THE
INNER
BEAUTY
BIBLE

'BEAUTY IS NOT IN THE FACE; BEAUTY IS A LIGHT IN THE HEART.'

Kahlil Gibran

THE INNER BEAUTY BIBLE

LAUREY SIMMONS

Thorsons

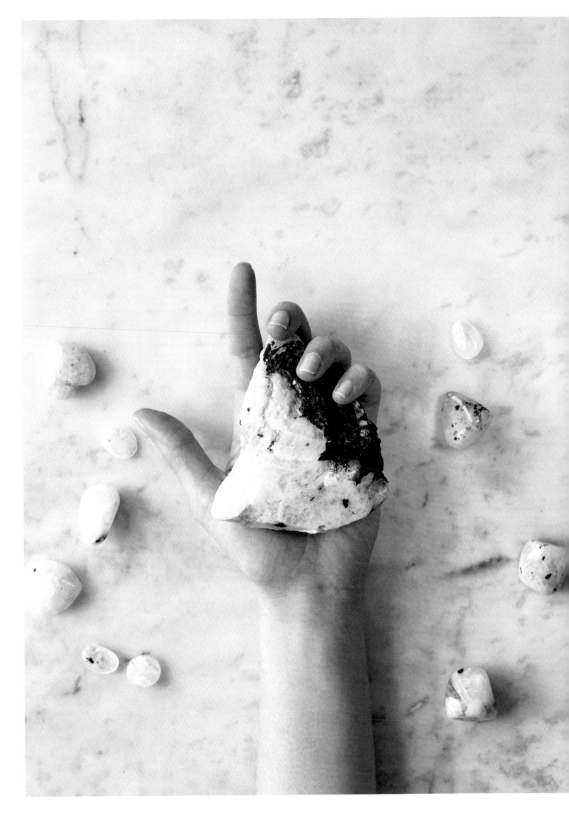

Contents

———————◇———————

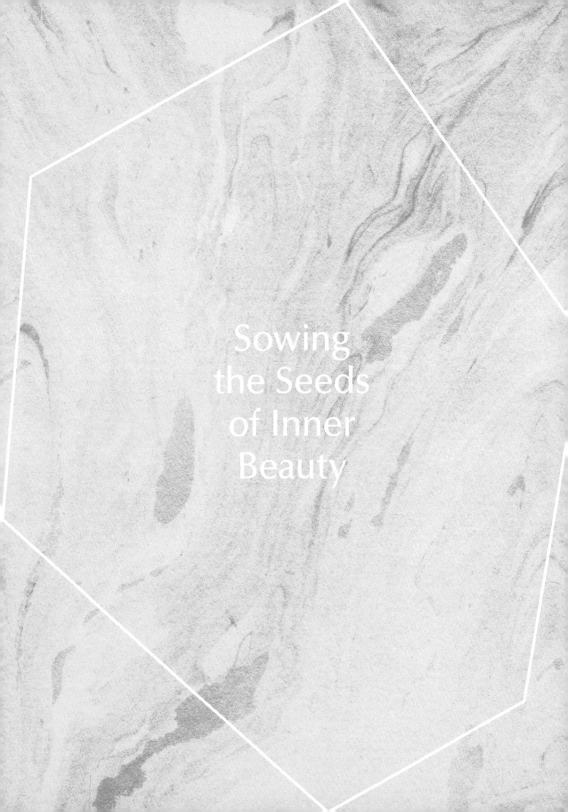

Sowing
the Seeds
of Inner
Beauty

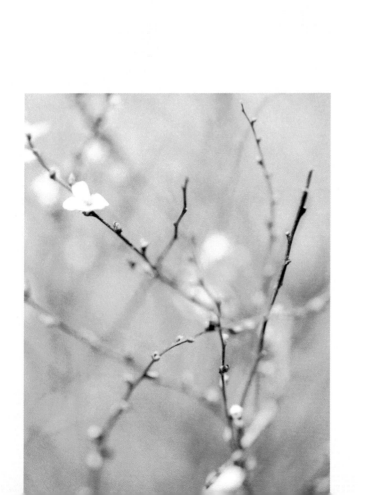
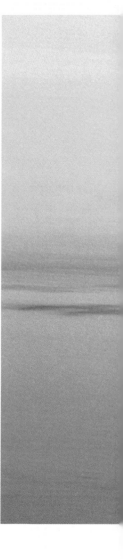

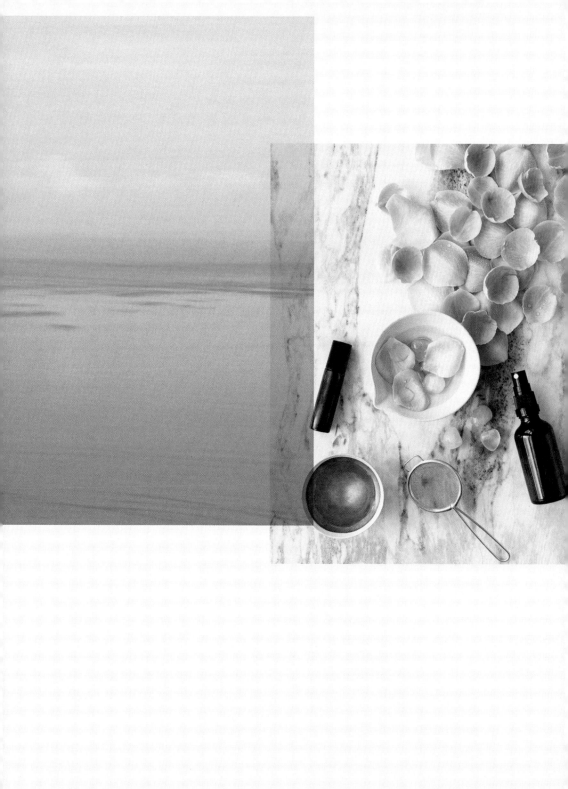

What is
Inner Beauty?

It's the surprise act of kindness from that man driving the bus.
It's the laughter of a friend who has suffered so much.
It's a giggling baby on an overcrowded train.
It's the fragrance of a rose, given freely again.
It's looking in the mirror and loving my soul.
It's embracing those changes, as we all grow old.
It's a long, loving hug that says 'we're in this together'.
It's the dawning truth when someone dies,
That life is precious,
And love is all that really matters in the end.

Inner Beauty is like a kaleidoscope: a beautiful way of seeing, with as many dimensions as there are eyes to see. The word kaleidoscope is actually derived from the Greek words *kalos* meaning 'beautiful' and *eidos* meaning 'that which is seen'. What kind of visions does the idea of Inner Beauty conjure up in your mind?

I've been immersed in the world of beauty for most of my career. Originally as a make-up artist in fashion and music, my job was to make people look more beautiful. But then I fell in love with crystals and sacred rituals, and my relationship with beauty deepened. Although I loved helping my clients feel amazing before their big event, I got to a point where I realized there was something missing. At the end of the day we all go home and wash our faces off, back to staring at our stripped-back selves. I realized there was a deeper kind of beauty that I could help myself and my clients connect to. I started to lay out crystals and other sacred objects next to the lipsticks and blushers in my make-up station. This simple act had such a lovely and calming effect on me, and on my clients, during what were often super-long and busy working days. I discovered that beautiful objects and sensory rituals can help us connect to an Inner Beauty that is always there, just waiting for us to remember. Do you have moments in your life where you use objects of beauty to bring you a deep sense of inner peace, love or joy?

When Hollywood star and humanitarian Audrey Hepburn was asked towards the end of her life to reveal her beauty secrets, she said: 'The beauty of a woman is not in a facial mole but true beauty in a woman is reflected in her soul.'

Can you think of anyone in your life who radiates that unmistakable quality of Inner Beauty? Someone in whose presence you feel instantly at home? What is it about these people, these moments, these encounters, that touch our hearts just so?

Just as I'd try to capture the essence of roses in water as a child, as an adult I've been discovering how to capture the essence of Inner Beauty. Trust me, there've been plenty of times in my life when I've felt far from radiant. But even in those more challenging moments of life, I've often felt like there is a voice that whispers to me, pointing me back to the beauty in my heart. Sometimes this whisper would come in the shape of a kind gesture or the scent of a flower; the simplest things that could in seconds wake me up from an irritable mood.

One of the most incredible phenomena of recent times has been the growth in mindfulness. It inspires me to see more and more people slowing down and tuning in to their inner worlds. A big part of mindfulness is bringing our attention away from our manic minds to our more grounded senses. For me, when we bring our attention to our senses, we allow ourselves to connect more deeply with the beauty of the world. When we slow down and connect with the beauty of the world through our senses, it opens up a greater space for the beauty inside ourselves. This is the sweet essence of the mindful rituals I am sharing with you in this book.

Of course, I totally get how it is being a busy bee in modern life, juggling work, home, relationships. Sometimes it's hard to remember to stop and smell the roses. We're exposed to such a whirlwind of media with hidden and not-so-hidden messages about how we should look, how we should feel and what we need to make us happy. The beauty industry is ever growing. And life is just becoming faster and faster. We find ourselves with an overwhelming sense of having loads to do and never enough time to do it. I know when I'm overwhelmed, I often feel like climbing into bed, snuggling up and switching off. I can easily get lost in the rabbit hole of mindless reality TV shows, gorging on comfort food, shrinking back into my shell. And there's absolutely nothing wrong with downtime; we definitely need downtime just to restore ourselves. But I've also realized it's life-enriching to find ways in our day-to-day life where we can simply slow down and re-connect to our Inner Beauty. In the middle of the storm of modern life, Inner Beauty is the stable eye. As we cultivate our Inner Beauty, we will be kinder to ourselves, and kinder to each other. We are all on a journey back to a place of beauty that's already there, a secret garden hidden inside all of us, just waiting to be rediscovered.

'I realized there was a deeper kind of beauty I could help myself and my clients connect to.'

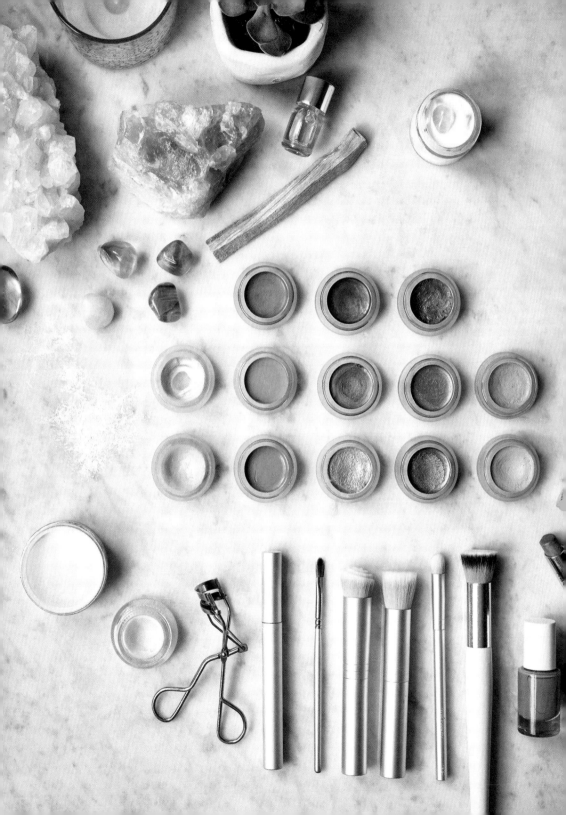

How to Use This Book

My hope in writing this book is to help you create beautiful sacred spaces and simple rituals that will strengthen your connection to Inner Beauty. Adding these flourishes of beauty to my own life, along with a clear, mindful intention, has repeatedly helped bring me back to a more positive, peaceful and loving space.

The book is divided into sections representing different aspects of your life. You'll get tips on how to incorporate rituals derived from ancient wisdom traditions into your modern life. You'll be able to turn to different pages in the book, according to your particular need in any given moment. You might think of this as a recipe book for Inner Beauty. Once you start to build these Inner Beauty rituals into your daily life, you will find that your connection to your Inner Beauty becomes more stable, and you will naturally start to see more beauty in the world around you. Wayne Dyer, a spiritual teacher who speaks directly to my heart, explained this process perfectly when he said: 'If you change the way you look at things, the things you look at change.'

In this chapter are some key ideas that I've found really helpful as I explore ever more deeply the world of Inner Beauty:

Inner and outer beauty are
two sides of the same coin.

Objects in the world around us affect
our inner world through our senses.

Our inner world is like a garden that needs certain
ingredients for beautiful things to grow.

Intention and attention together
make magic happen.

1. INNER AND OUTER BEAUTY ARE TWO SIDES OF THE SAME COIN

This first idea is really the most important of all. It's all too easy to become fixated on the external appearance of things, especially ourselves. How many days do we wake up in the morning, look in the mirror and find something about our appearance that we dislike, affecting our confidence for the rest of the day? When we start the day with a self-critical mind, we feel a bit rubbish inside and it doesn't matter how much make-up we put on, we'll still be a less beautiful being in the world. On the other hand, if we look after our Inner Beauty by cultivating certain important qualities like self-compassion, patience, forgiveness, we'll instantly become more attractive in the world. Inner Beauty radiates in such a powerful way that we appear more beautiful in the eyes of others. In the same way, if we treat ourselves like the goddesses we are, looking after our external appearance in a less critical, more sacred, kind and loving way, then we'll naturally radiate that unmistakable light of Inner Beauty. Inner and outer beauty really do go hand in hand.

2. OBJECTS IN THE WORLD AROUND US AFFECT OUR INNER WORLD THROUGH OUR SENSES

We are gifted with senses. Our senses are windows into a world filled with beauty. Just as we need to give nourishment to our body, we also need to nourish our soul; and the most powerful way for me is through my senses. Sometimes when I slow down to smell the blossom on a tree, it's like all the day's worry and fear, all the doubts and insecurities just evaporate from my being. When I stop to gaze at a beautiful old tree, it grounds me and fills me with gratitude for Nature and life itself. My love for crystals is more than anything else grown from my appreciation of their visual beauty. Any time we tune our senses in to perceiving beauty in the world, whether it's a stunning piece of music, the smell of a rose, a beautiful stone or a piece of art, we are awakening the Inner Beauty of our soul.

Each of our senses can transform us in a totally unique way. Our eyes, as they say, are the windows to our soul, and these windows can function in quite miraculous ways. An amazing study was carried out in the 1970s on patients recovering from gallbladder surgery.[1] Even though gallbladder surgery is very routine, for some reason, certain patients were recovering much faster than others. When researchers looked into this pattern, they discovered that some of the hospital rooms faced on to a brick wall, whilst others faced on to a row of beautiful trees. Guess what … it was the patients looking at the trees who recovered faster every time. This same kind of effect has been demonstrated with colours (pink repeatedly makes people less aggressive), with shapes (rounded edges tend to make people feel more peaceful), and with objects (the presence of a briefcase in a room tends to make people more competitive). Now, many of us can't look at trees all day, but we can surround ourselves with beautiful objects from the natural world that have the power to restore us. Have a think now – what natural objects might awaken a real feeling of joy inside you?

Our sense of touch can really affect our emotional state. Have you ever worn a cardigan that was a bit itchy and made you feel irritable all day? Did you have one security object when you were younger that you just had to take with you everywhere? Even from a young age, we seem to understand that holding certain objects can make us feel certain ways. We can even see this influence of touch in our language, for example when we say, 'I am having a rough day.' For me, something magical happens when I hold and interact with objects such as crystals in a mindful way.

Helen Keller described smell as a 'potent wizard that transports you across thousands of miles and all the years you have lived'. I really love those words, as smell really does have a magical effect on me, and I'm sure on you. Studies have shown that the smell of baking cookies makes people more likely to help a stranger. Isn't that amazing! As we get into the rituals in this book, I'll be suggesting different smells, incenses and oils that act as magical reminders of our Inner Beauty qualities.

The last sense for us to explore is hearing. Now, if you live in an urban environment like me then you'll probably be exposed to certain sounds that don't exactly help to make you feel peaceful. The honking of horns, the neighbour's dog barking all night, whatever it is, sounds in built-up environments can sometimes have a very negative effect on how we feel. This is because our ears are directly linked to our nervous systems in quite a powerful way. The vagus nerve, which is the channel through which the love hormone oxytocin is released in our body, connects our ears to every organ in our body. On the plus side, this means that soothing sounds (like melodies sung to a baby) release oxytocin into our system. The important thing to remember is that we can create sounds, even in small apartments in super-busy cities, that will help to relax our nervous system and can awaken beautiful qualities within us. In many indigenous traditions, sound, sacred singing and drums are all used in ceremonies as medicine to heal. Have a think now: what is the go-to song that you listen to when your heart needs some TLC? How does that song make you feel on the inside?

3. OUR INNER WORLD IS LIKE A GARDEN THAT NEEDS CERTAIN INGREDIENTS FOR BEAUTIFUL THINGS TO GROW

It inspires me to see more and more people really taking time to look after their inner world, with crystals, meditation, rituals. I like to use the metaphor of a garden for our inner world. Just like a garden, if we don't give enough attention to the plant life, cutting away any dead branches, making sure the plants are getting enough water and sun, then the plants don't grow in a healthy way. It's just the same with our Inner Beauty. I know when I find the time to nourish my Inner Beauty, then qualities like kindness, gratitude and forgiveness have more chance of growing. I've already talked about using beautiful objects to reflect back beauty. But the truth is, we can't always surround ourselves with beauty. Sometimes it's necessary that we carry that sense of beauty into a situation that might be very challenging, where we don't have all our crystals, our flowers, our nice hot bath ritual to help us reconnect. We'll look at how to nourish Inner Beauty qualities in more detail as we go through the book. For now, it's good just to acknowledge that if we regularly give nourishment to our inner world, it can continue to grow and spread its beautiful light, even when the sky is full of dark clouds.

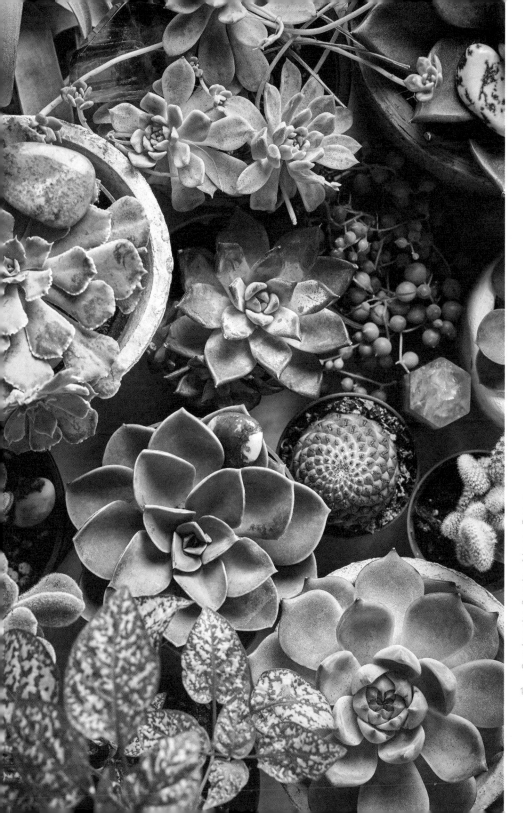

Sowing the Seeds of Inner Beauty

4. INTENTION AND ATTENTION TOGETHER MAKE MAGIC HAPPEN

I grew up in a Jewish family and was surrounded by rituals. But to be honest, at some stage in my life I lost touch a little with the real value of these rituals. Although I could always appreciate the beauty of lighting candles on a Friday night, standing next to my mum as she marked the beginning of the Sabbath with a graceful, welcoming gesture of her hands waving over the candle-flames, after a certain age I feel like I disconnected from the real magic of ritual. It was only in the last few years that I've started to appreciate in a different way the two factors that together have the power to make rituals so magical: intention and attention. You see, when we do most routine activities in our day-to-day lives, we tend to have distracted minds. When I brush my teeth, for example, I often find myself planning my route to a meeting, thinking about emails I need to respond to, etc. But when I'm practising mindful rituals, it gives me a chance to slow everything down, quieten my mind, and consciously decide how I want to be that day. Rituals guide us gracefully out of our auto-pilot mode, creating a magical space where something more beautiful can emerge.

Wayne Dyer wrote so much about the power of intention. His philosophy could be summed up really simply in this one quote of his: 'our intention creates our reality'. Intention to me simply means setting out a crystal-clear plan in my mind of how I want to be and what outcome I hope for in a situation. So often we don't do this, and our minds and bodies default to our unconscious intentions, those old beliefs we carry from childhood that are often limiting and don't serve our Highest Self. How often in your average day do you set a crystal-clear intention of how you want to be before engaging in an activity? When we set a clear intention and cultivate positive feelings so that our whole body is signed up to this intention, we can reverse our unconscious habits and influence our reality in quite miraculous ways.

It can be relatively easy to set an intention (just think of New Year's resolutions), but if our mind gets regularly distracted then the intention will never be able to manifest. There have been so many times when I set an intention in the morning, to be kind, to be more patient, more loving, and then I have a million and one messages, phone calls, emails, to-do-lists and after an hour or so and an encounter with a moody shopkeeper, it's like I've completely and utterly lost track of my intention. This is where attention, the ability to keep bringing our minds back to that one important thing, is so important. In mindfulness meditation, it doesn't matter how many times your mind wanders off, it's the practice of bringing your attention back again and again that really has the biggest impact. The same thing applies to intentions and Inner Beauty rituals. It doesn't matter how many times we might get distracted during the day, if we can notice our distracted mind and bring our attention back time and again to that Inner Beauty quality we want to manifest, then we're very likely going to start seeing changes quite soon. Attention does require discipline, but it's worth the effort.

'Rituals guide
us gracefully out
of our auto-pilot
mode, creating
a magical space
where something
more beautiful
can emerge.'

My Story

There's something magical about the smell of roses. Often when I smell a rose, I'm transported instantly back to myself as a young girl. I remember endless summer days spent picking rose petals from our garden; losing myself in a dreamy world of smell, colour and abundant life. I would ever so mindfully put the roses in bottles of water and try to sell my potions outside our house. Looking back now, I can really appreciate how naturally I was drawn to the beauty of these sensory rituals. Can you remember connecting with the beauty of Nature as a child? Can you remember the things you loved to pick, to hold, to make? Can you remember how simple things like colour, sound and smell made you feel? Building outdoor dens, making daisy-chains, picking buttercups and holding them under a friend's chin.

How to make a rosewater spritzer

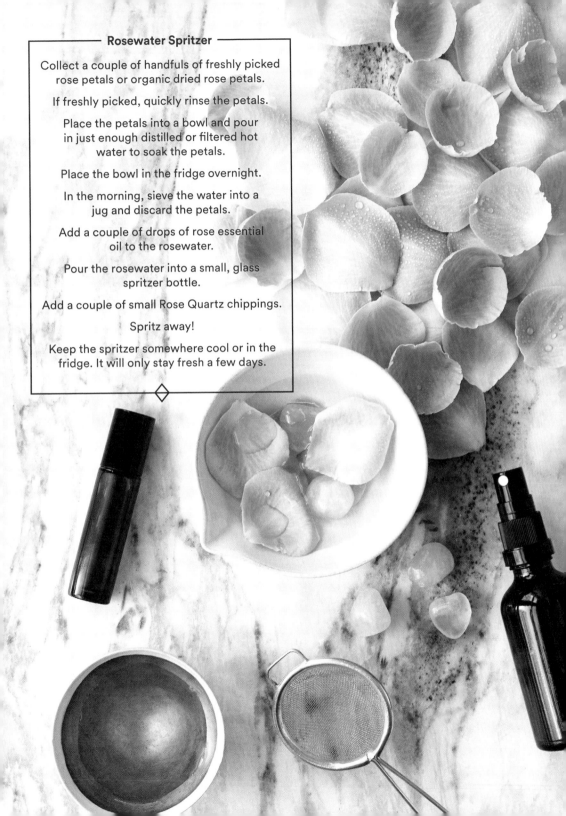

Rosewater Spritzer

Collect a couple of handfuls of freshly picked rose petals or organic dried rose petals.

If freshly picked, quickly rinse the petals.

Place the petals into a bowl and pour in just enough distilled or filtered hot water to soak the petals.

Place the bowl in the fridge overnight.

In the morning, sieve the water into a jug and discard the petals.

Add a couple of drops of rose essential oil to the rosewater.

Pour the rosewater into a small, glass spritzer bottle.

Add a couple of small Rose Quartz chippings.

Spritz away!

Keep the spritzer somewhere cool or in the fridge. It will only stay fresh a few days.

Like the petals of the rose, my childhood connection to beauty unfolded in so many different directions. I had a real passion for art from a young age. I got really inspired by artists like Georgia O'Keeffe, whose work would speak directly to that place of beauty inside my heart. I channelled this energy into my own art. I could spend months working on one painting, completely focussed on the intricate details, often of flowers, shells or stones. Painting became a real heart-expanding meditation for me. As the saying goes, 'love is in the detail'. I think this pretty much sums up how I approach most things in life.

Some of my most precious childhood memories are of walking the beaches of Mallorca with my mum, looking for the prettiest pebbles, just feeling a sense of wonder, even at this young age, for the beauty of Mother Nature and her magical powers. We'd bring these pebbles home and place them on my Grandmother's gravestone. This ritual is an ancient Jewish practice; in the Kabbalah, the soul is said to be carved from the stone of a mountain, and so the placement of stones on a grave is an invitation, welcoming the soul of the departed to come down and rest upon the tombstones during a visit.

But even at times in my life when things definitely weren't so rosy, there was something inside me, something magnetically drawing me to the beauty of the world, that continued to unfold. I remember buying my first spiritual book, called *The Seat of the Soul* by Gary Zukav, after watching an interview with him on Oprah Winfrey. I guess this was the first step into my own 'adult' spiritual path. I'm laughing now, remembering the first time I tried to meditate. I was about sixteen years old, sitting on my bed, just waiting, waiting, waiting for something to happen ... but with one eye open! Looking back I really appreciate the innocent way in which I was searching for something deeper.

The love of beauty and sacred ritual magically wove its way into my adult life. I became a make-up artist, moved to London from Leeds and began assisting celebrity make-up artist Mary Greenwell. I soon created my own career as a make-up artist in the fashion and music industries. Putting on make-up can of course be a kind of ritual in itself. There is something meditative about it, the attention to detail, the repetition, the time for self-care. And so, as I developed more of an interest in crystals, meditation and conscious living, my approach to my make-up work naturally evolved. I started to create little sacred spaces for my clients, using crystals, essential oils and meditation, which seemed to add a deeper, more sacred dimension to the make-up ritual. My clients started to tell me that they experienced a kind of peacefulness and inner joy that had a real, positive impact on them before their shoot or big event. This new sacred dimension I was bringing to the beauty process was especially helpful and grounding to myself and clients when we were on the road. As we'd travel from city to city, and from country to country on music tours, I'd bring a portable sacred space with crystals and oils, and even got some of the band wearing crystal necklaces to bring good energy on stage. All of these rituals really helped us to ground ourselves and re-connect to a space of stillness in the midst of busy tour life.

Inspired by this growing connection to Inner Beauty in my life as a make-up artist, I started to look deeper into beauty rituals and became especially interested in crystals as a tool for Inner Beauty. I discovered to my delight that crushed crystals like Malachite and Lapis Lazuli were used in Ancient Egypt as sacred make-up mineral blends for living goddesses. Just imagine for a moment what kind of a sense of beauty might have existed at this time, if people were consciously adding spiritual materials into their beauty products. People have clearly recognized for a long time that nurturing beauty is not an exercise in vanity, but an essential process to keep you closer to the divine.

As I look back, I can now see the universe has been guiding me along my spiritual path, and this path has been lined with crystals. I first became interested in crystals during a difficult time in my life. I was feeling quite down emotionally, I'd just had a flare-up of Crohn's (an inflammatory auto-immune condition of the stomach), and I was seeking extra support and self-healing. I started going for crystal healing myself. I remember my first ever healing session, entering the sacred space and feeling the energy of all the beautiful crystals laid out before me. I was immediately transported to that same place of tranquil beauty and inner peace I had felt on the beach as a child collecting pebbles. And so, my love affair with crystals was born.

When I met my husband Louis, my spiritual journey was accelerated. He was running a therapeutic education provision at the time, teaching meditation and providing therapy to troubled teenagers from London. We soon realized a wonderful way for us to combine our passions would be to set up a meditation group, where Louis would lead the meditations and I would bring the shanti vibes with my crystals, oils and singing bowls. The friends who came to these groups really seemed to find a deeper sense of connection and meaning in the sacred space and ritual we were offering.

After we got married, we took a sabbatical travelling around India, starting our journey in Kerala and meandering our way North. Mother India really blew my heart wide open. I remember feelings of awe and joy at the rainbow of colours, the smells of incense on every corner, the exquisite textiles and jewellery. I was touched by the fact that India has proudly held on to this sacred knowledge for thousands of years, using beautiful objects, smells and colours to keep people connected to that place of Inner Beauty. During our adventure, we immersed ourselves with the local culture, staying with Indian families and experiencing first-hand daily rituals, religious festivals and ceremonies, where we learned how spirituality and a sense of the sacred was ingrained in so many aspects of daily life. In Pushkar, we became friends with a beautiful spiritual teacher, Jaggu, who had a very simple ashram built around a Banyan tree on the edge of the holy lake. In this small space, he would simply share his wisdom and love freely as he sat by a sacred fire that was kept going twenty-four hours a day. Around this fire, in this very humble space, there would always be laid out beautiful flowers, oils and incense. To celebrate this spirit of beauty and sacred ritual, I started to collect the most beautiful things I found. This was where the seed of The Colourful Dot came into bloom. My vision for this online shop was to create a space to help nourish that precious and sacred connection between inner and outer beauty, stocking crystals, sacred oils and other inspiring objects to be used in creating sacred spaces and Inner Beauty rituals.

My appreciation for sacred ritual deepened whilst on a mountain pilgrimage with wisdom-keepers around Peru and Bolivia. I had the great honour of travelling with indigenous elders from the Q'ero, Quechua, Ayumara and Chumash tribes. In these indigenous cultures, rituals aren't something we do just to gain personal benefit, but are above all a way of showing deep gratitude and respect for Pachamama (Mother Earth). The one idea that really stuck in my heart was *ayni*, the native Andean concept that describes the 'sacred exchange' or reciprocity that is so vitally important, because we are all connected to each other by living energy. When we saw the Winter Solstice sun rise from the top of a sacred mountain on the Isla del Sol, the local people spontaneously opened their hearts to us, sharing songs and food, and we returned this spontaneous gifting with our own songs and gifts. This was *ayni* in action. This period in my life deepened my understanding that everything, from the earth we walk upon, to the pebbles we find on the beach, to the water we bathe in, has a unique spirit that is in constant exchange with the world. Did you know that peace lilies not only give us oxygen but they also remove toxins such as benzene and ammonia from the air? We honour the beauty and generosity of this spirit, in Nature and inside of ourselves (we are after all Nature), through reciprocity and ritual.

As I look to the path ahead, I feel so thankful to be on this journey. The more I learn through my own study and practice, the more I realize how important it is to come back to that Inner Beauty space of kindness, gratitude and love. And coming back to that space is a never-ending practice, one I definitely still struggle with some days. But no matter how far from the path we stray, the next day is always a chance for a fresh start. I really hope you find this book connects with you on some level. Even if you just take away one single idea or practice that inspires you to shine your light more brightly upon the world, then that will be enough.

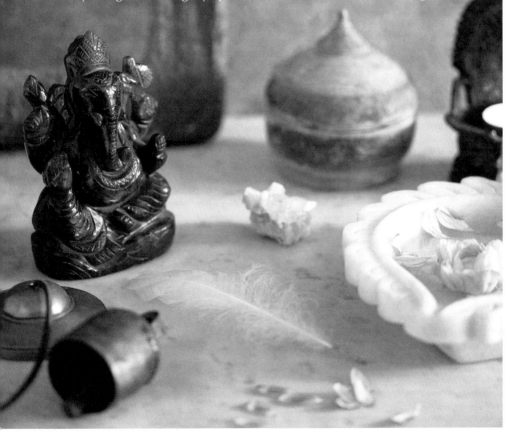

Sowing the Seeds of Inner Beauty

A Very Short History
of Beauty and Ritual

Beauty and ritual belong together. Ritual without a sense of beauty is merely routine.

Imagine for a moment your daily routine of travelling into work. How often do you connect with the beauty around you or within you? I think for most of us, our commute to work is just a means of getting from A to B. We're mostly focussed on the destination and rarely on the journey. An amazing experiment was carried out by a world-famous violinist called Joshua Bell.[2] He spent a day in a subway station in Washington DC performing some of the most beautiful pieces of music ever composed. Hardly anyone stopped to tune in, apart from one young girl who slowed down to listen, until her mum hurriedly dragged her along. The conclusion of the study was that when we're stuck in mindless routine, when we're purely focussed on the destination, we miss out on the beauty that is available to us in everyday situations.

It's incredible to think that our earliest ancestors, going back a hundred thousand years, managed to find the time to mark and appreciate beauty despite living with much greater, more real risk then we do today. A Stone Age burial site discovered in France contained two women who had been buried in a ritual way with beautiful snail shell necklaces. The amazing thing about this discovery is that the beauty of the necklaces has endured all this time.

In Ancient Greece, the concept of beauty was central to life, but it was quite clear that beauty referred not just to how you look, but equally to beautiful actions; how we act in the world can be beautiful and contribute to the highest good. The Greek word for beautiful, *kalos*, means both aesthetically beautiful and virtuous.

Many indigenous cultures have for a long time understood the sacred connection between inner and outer beauty, which they channel into the world through prayer, dance, arts, ritual and ceremony. Navajo Indians have a concept I'm totally in love with, called 'The Beauty Way'. The Beauty Way is a philosophy for life, the main focus of which is to appreciate and maintain the beauty in the world around us and in the world within us. Most importantly, beauty isn't just aesthetics; it is also the qualities we cultivate inside ourselves. The Beauty Way blessing is:

> *Shil hózhó*, 'with me there is beauty';
> *Shii' hózhó*, 'in me there is beauty';
> *Shaa hózhó*, 'from me beauty radiates'.

Take a moment to read over these statements and really let them sink in. When I allow my heart to connect to the ancient wisdom contained in these blessings, I'm filled with inspiration and hope. In The Beauty Way tradition, whenever someone feels out of harmony with life or in need of some TLC, they're given 'medicine' in the form of beautiful ceremonies, performed by the tribe just to reconnect that person to their sense of beauty. In these Beauty Way ceremonies, songs would be sung and sandpaintings created, all for the specific purpose of healing the 'patient'. And the 'patient' would participate in all of this, singing the songs, and even actually getting into the sandpainting to bring the healing to an end. This is how Gary Witherspoon, an expert in Native American culture, describes the spirit of this ceremony: 'The sandpainting is not just to be seen but also to be absorbed, its beauty and harmony heal mind and body.'

Imagine that! Every time you feel out of sorts, your loved ones surround you and sing beautiful songs, make beautiful art for you and say beautiful blessings for you (with me there is beauty), and your only responsibility is to accept the beauty being showered upon you (in me there is beauty), so that you can go back out into the world and shine your light (from me beauty radiates). Without consciously planning it, I was already weaving aspects of the Beauty Way in the meditation groups I held with my husband. By creating a beautiful space for friends to connect and be really open with one another, rather than the usual chit-chat we tend to engage in in our rushed daily lives, we all experienced a sense of great heart-opening and healing, as well as a stronger sense of community, helping each other to focus on what is most important to us, on how we want to be in the world.

One aspect of beauty and ritual that can be seen throughout history is the celebration of the wild beauty of Nature. These traditions often refer to Nature as a maternal figure, giver of life and nourishment: in Native American tradition we have Mother Earth, and Pachamama is the name of Mother Earth in ancient Incan wisdom. As I experienced in Peru, rituals around Mother Nature are a means to give something back to her (food, tobacco, sweets) as a token of appreciation. I love these traditions and how they contrast with the Modern way in which we have tended for some time to just take from Mother Earth without reciprocating.

A deep respect for the feminine beauty and power of nature underpins many such rituals. Nature is wild. She can sometimes appear serene, peaceful, flowing, and at other times she can appear angry and destructive. But there is a beauty in her cycles that I think should be celebrated. The key here is the cycles. Just think of the waxing and waning of the moon, or the ebb and flow of the tides. There is a great peace that can be found in accepting the cycles of our life, and so letting go of the idea that we should be aiming always to be more: more happy, more full of energy, more giving. As the biblical verse (Ecclesiastes 5:7) reminds us: 'There is a time to plant and a time to uproot … a time to scatter stones and a time to gather them.'

Beyond the cycles of Mother Earth overall, individual plants, trees and animals in the natural world have been seen in many indigenous traditions as having a spirit we can ask for protection from through ritual. In the Celtic tradition (Celts are the indigenous people of Britain), every mountain, river, tree, plant, animal or rock had a spirit which would be worshipped. The spirits of water were particularly respected as givers and sustainers of life, and healing rituals would be performed at natural springs. It is said that the River Thames that runs through London gets its name from the Celtic goddess Tamesis.

Even though we may think today that some of these ancient beliefs seem a bit far-out, conjuring the stereotype of the tree-hugging hippy, we can all instinctively appreciate the healing power of Nature. For those of us who live in cities, we instinctively know that when we're in need of rejuvenation we take ourselves off to the countryside, to the forests, to the seaside. There's just something about being in nature, about appreciating the beauty of nature, including the beauty of our own nature, that really lifts our spirits and restores a sense of balance to our hearts and minds. When we're in Nature, we can stop clock-watching, detox from our devices, clear our minds, slow down and get inspired. The eternal beauty of Nature gets captured most perfectly by the Romantic poet John Keats, whose now famous lines read: 'To see a world in a grain of sand, and heaven in a wild flower. Hold infinity in the palms of your hand, and eternity in an hour.'

One of the lessons that Nature teaches me is that things can be beautiful, even though they're not 'perfect'. And Japanese tradition has developed a stunningly simple way in which we can celebrate the imperfect beauty of our own Nature. The concept is called *wabi-sabi*. The words refer to 'the wisdom and beauty of imperfection' (Taro Gold). One of my favourite examples of *wabi-sabi* is the Japanese tea ceremony, where utensils are purposefully chosen because they are simple, rustic, asymmetrical, and sometimes even deliberately chipped. But it was the way in which these imperfect objects were used with such great care, mindful grace and appreciation that brought the sense of beauty into the tea ritual.

These days we can get caught up in a drive to make things ever more perfect. I can see how easily the modern woman in particular can get weighed down with expectations to be a super-woman: being a perfect mum, a perfect wife or partner, a perfect friend, a perfect career woman, and the whole time trying to look good too. To nourish the inner garden that is our Inner Beauty, we can learn a lot from our ancestors and how they taught us to slow down, to turn our careful attention to the beautiful, especially in Nature, to look for the beautiful in everything, even or especially in those things that might seem imperfect at first glance. Life is not perfect. We will all at some point in our lives experience chips or cracks in the delicate china of our selves. Rather than brushing these imperfections under the carpet in a race to some perfect end goal, ancient wisdom traditions show us how we can embrace these cracks and see the beauty shining through them.

Sowing the Seeds of Inner Beauty

Defining Your Own
Inner Beauty

'The problem is you're afraid to acknowledge your
own beauty. Well, enough already. I sit before you
because I see your beauty, even if you don't.'

◇

Ram Dass

Before we get into the specific Inner Beauty rituals I've collected for you
here, I'd just like to kickstart our journey with a little ritual. This exercise
will help you to understand what Inner Beauty means to you. Whatever
you discover in this exercise will be your guide as you continue to cultivate
the beauty within.

First, it can really help if you get a journal that you can dedicate completely
to your own Inner Beauty. This can be a source of personal inspiration to you.
You can keep quotes that inspire you, images that invoke Inner Beauty qualities
for you, beautiful leaves you've collected. You can also write in here your answers
to some of the questions I will be asking you throughout the book. In this journal,
write down on the first page the following title: 'Inner Beauty to me is … '

Now, put down your pen for just a moment. It can help to close your eyes for
this exercise. Take in a deep breath and, with a big sigh, breathe out any stress or
tension. Bring to your mind an image of a beautiful flower. Notice what it looks
like, what colour it is, what it smells like, what it makes you feel inside. Now you've
connected to a space of Inner Beauty, allow into your mind's eye someone in your

life who has an abundance of Inner Beauty. This might be someone you know. It might equally be someone you've never met. It could be someone you've read about. It could even be a fictional character, a hero or heroine, a god or goddess, a spiritual teacher, or an everyday person who just has that luminescent quality. Trust the image that your mind offers you. As this example of Inner Beauty crystallizes in your mind's eye, take your time to explore what exactly it is about this person that brings for you an association with Inner Beauty. What are the qualities they represent for you? Are they kind, compassionate, grateful, light-hearted, forgiving, generous, serene, graceful, nurturing or something else? What are the specific gestures they made, the actions they took that represent Inner Beauty for you? Now allow yourself to sense what it feels like to be in their presence. What do you feel, and where do you feel it in your body? Perhaps you notice a certain warmth in your heart, a smile in your mind, or just a sense of peace or of being at home. Whatever the feeling is, allow yourself to really get to know this feeling for a moment. This is your feeling of Inner Beauty.

When you feel you have explored this Inner Beauty image in as much detail as you need, write down the qualities that you recognized in this person. Beneath or next to this, write down some words to describe the feelings that this example of Inner Beauty conjured up for you.

Now have a look through this list, and see if there's anything else you'd add to it that you'd associate with Inner Beauty. If you're feeling creative, you can draw something that represents Inner Beauty, or decorate the page with beautiful things, like pressed flowers or pretty fabrics.

This page will serve you as your reminder. You can turn to it whenever you're feeling disconnected from your own Inner Beauty. You can even put it in your sacred space.

Kindness

Patience

Compassion

Forgiveness

Grace

Generosity

Gratitude

Humility

Courage

Confidence

Honesty

Love

INNER BEAUTY QUALITIES

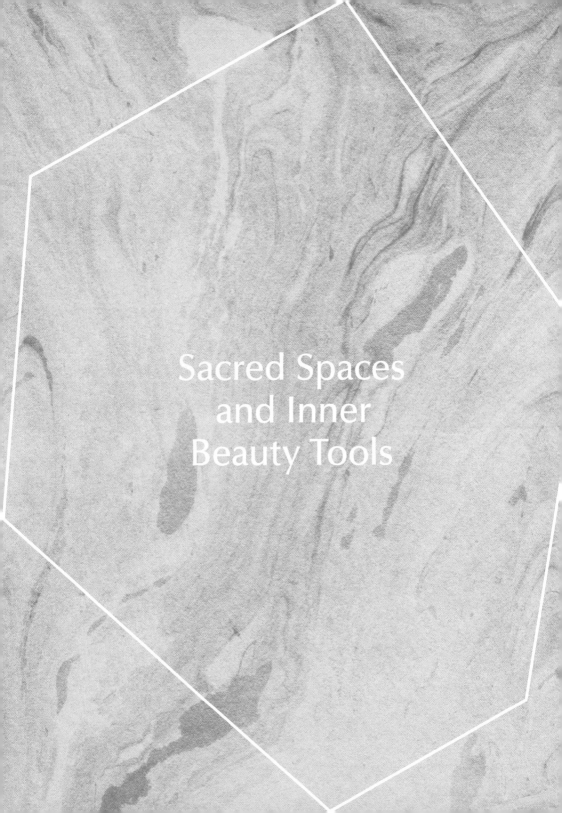

Sacred Spaces
and Inner
Beauty Tools

2

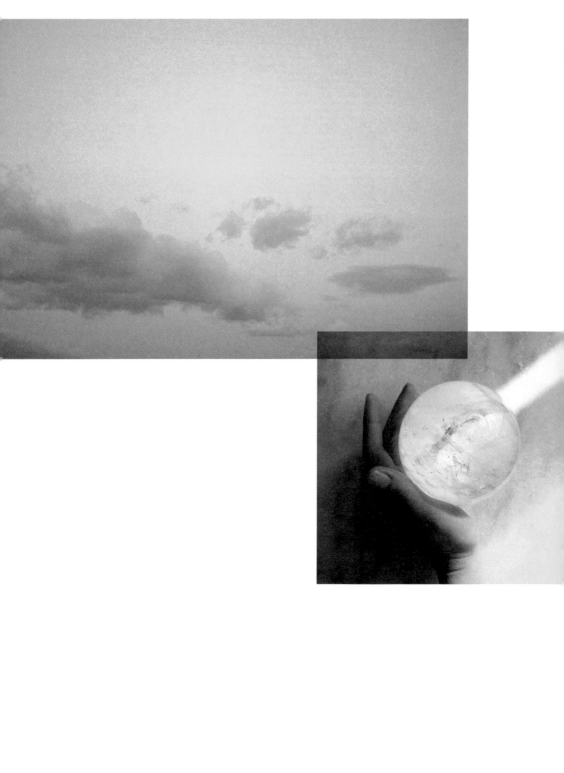

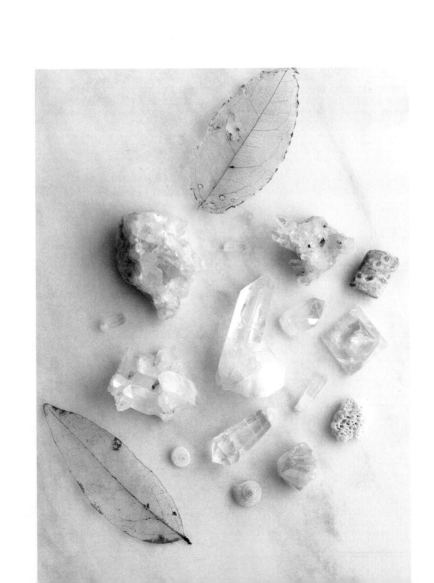

A Sacred Space
Is a Gift to Your Soul

'A sacred space is where you can find
yourself over and over again.'

Joseph Campbell

A sacred space is simply one corner of our home environment where we keep beautiful objects that are special or sacred to us. Keeping a sacred space is a precious gift to our soul, a mirror reflecting back to us our Inner Beauty. Whenever I feel off-track, the sacred beauty of this space helps to refocus my mind and heart, a lovely reminder of how I want to be in the world.

You don't need to be religious or spiritual to have a sacred space. All you need is a desire in your heart to be the best person you can be. One of the greatest challenges in life is to remember how we want to be in the world. I know for myself that, even with my best intentions to be calm, centred and beautiful on the inside, life can at times be overwhelming and I simply forget, finding myself worrying about the growing inbox I need to respond to, the to-do list that never gets any smaller. Jonathan Z. Smith describes a sacred space as being like a 'focussing lens'. The nice thing about a sacred space is that, once you've set it up in a way that feels right for you, it will support you for as long as it remains there and it will make your heart sing with joy, so you will be magnetically drawn to it every day.

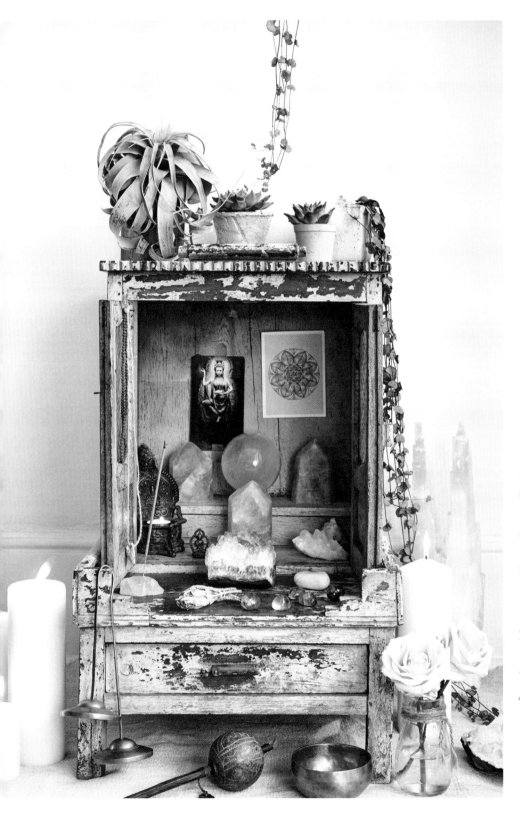

Setting up Your Sacred Space

'Some people look for a beautiful place,
others make a place beautiful.'

Hazrat Inayat Khan (Sufi Master)

FINDING THE SPACE

To make a sacred space, you first need to decide on one place in your home where you can regularly spend time without too much distraction. You might want to consider finding a place that you will naturally see on a daily basis. Even if you just walk past it and get a glimpse of the beautiful reminders there, sometimes that's all you need. But it does need to be out of the way enough, so that the objects you lay down won't need to be moved.

To find the right spot for your sacred space, set aside some time to walk around your house and get a sense from both a practical level and a heartfelt level of where you feel the space needs to be. It helps to choose your sacred space if you can do this at a time when you feel relatively calm. Remember, a sacred space is one of the greatest gifts you can give to yourself, so, as you move through this process, allow your heart to open with a sense of loving tenderness towards yourself.

Before you walk around your space, take a moment to stand in one place and imagine that tree-like roots are connecting your body to the earth and that you are being supported, grounded and nourished. When you feel ready, simply take your time to walk around and identify the one place you'll be able to hang out in whenever you need that Inner Beauty boost.

Once you've found your perfect spot, the next step is to cleanse the unwanted energy that may be in this place. Have you ever walked into a room and felt an uncomfortable sensation even though nobody was there? Emotional and spiritual energies can be left in a place; they can reside in material objects like floorboards and furniture and can even linger in the air. This is why many ancient traditions use cleansing to purify the energy in spaces. Some tools with which you can cleanse your sacred space include sound, herbs, oils and certain woods. We'll look in more detail at energy cleansing tools a little later.

CHOOSING OBJECTS FOR YOUR SACRED SPACE

Once you've found and cleansed this place, the next step is to choose the objects that will come together to make your space truly sacred. The best objects to use are those that have a special meaning for you, those that help to remind you of your highest qualities – like compassion, creativity, peace and love. Before buying anything, I recommend taking a mindful look around your home or garden, just to see what things you already have. It's important that you're in a peaceful headspace and connected to your heart before you walk around, as it's only from this place that sacred objects will call out to you clearly. Maybe you have some objects that you brought back from a special day or a special trip, like pretty shells from a beach or a souvenir from a special moment? As you walk around on your sacred treasure hunt, keep these questions in mind when you consider objects: what feelings, thoughts or sensations does this object evoke for me? Are these feelings, thoughts or sensations something I want to have more of in my life? If the answer to the second question is a definite 'YES', then this object could be a perfect companion for your sacred space. Don't worry if you can't find anything obvious in your home, as you look through the different Inner Beauty tools in this chapter, you'll get more of a sense of what kind of things might work best for you. You can definitely find lots of inspiration online too, or on my @thecolourfuldot Instagram page.

CREATING AND NURTURING YOUR SACRED SPACE

Creating your sacred space is a meditation in itself. When I arrange the objects in my own sacred space, it's a form of sacred art. And making my sacred space look beautiful always makes me feel more beautiful on the inside. When you're happy with your own sacred art-piece, it's a good idea to set a general intention for the space. What one single quality would you most like to be reminded of every time you check in with this space? It might be that you want this space to remind you to be peaceful or loving or forgiving. Whatever it is for you, you can write down your general intention on a small piece of paper and leave this on display in your sacred space.

But, creating the sacred space is really just the beginning. Once it's created, I find it really helps to nurture this space on a regular basis. Remember, your sacred space is a garden for growing your inner goddess. For some tips on how to nurture your sacred space, turn to page 92.

Sacred Space Meditation

I love spending time in my sacred space. The great thing about hanging out in a beautiful sacred space is that it makes meditation easy: sometimes I just leave my eyes open and let the beauty before me cheer up my soul. Sometimes, I'll take in hand one of the objects from my sacred space and use that as the focus of my meditation. So if I'm feeling the need to nurture my heart, I'll take a Rose Quartz crystal in my hand (Rose Quartz is associated with love), close my eyes and gently bring my attention to follow my breath. As I breathe in, I bring the word 'love' to mind and feel my heart expanding and I visualize my body filling out from the centre with a soft pink light. As I breathe out, I imagine breathing out unwanted energy.

If you are the sort of person who finds the idea of formal meditation a bit too full-on, then no need to fear. The very act of creating and regularly nurturing your sacred space is honestly an amazing meditation in itself. The most important thing about sacred spaces is that they're a window to your Highest Self, your inner goddess. As long as you keep polishing these windows, you will be able to find yourself over and over again.

Tools to Use in
Your Sacred Space

CRYSTALS

A Brief History of Crystals

Although the idea of crystals for some might conjure up visions of long-haired, flower-powered hippies getting their woo-woo on, crystals have actually been celebrated in many different civilizations and cultures for thousands of years. This is not surprising. When you hold a crystal in your hand for the first time, you cannot help but be touched by the magical beauty of these gifts from Mother Earth. Even as far back as biblical times, we see the beauty of crystals celebrated. In the Old Testament Book of Ezekiel we're told:

> You were in Eden, the garden of God; every precious stone was
> your covering: the ruby, the topaz and the diamond; the beryl, the
> onyx and the jasper; the lapis lazuli, the turquoise and the emerald
> … on the day that you were created, they were prepared.

I just love the idea that crystals have been our steady companions throughout the whole of human history. They were collected not just for their rarity but also for their healing properties, as we can see in this quote from an ancient mystical Jewish text, called the Baba Batra:

> Abraham had a precious stone hung round his neck which brought immediate healing to any sick person who looked on it, and when Abraham our father left this world, the Blessed Holy One hung it from the wheel of the sun.

The word 'crystal' actually derives from the Greek word *'krustallos'* meaning ice. The story goes that when the Greeks came across Quartz in the mountains they believed it to be eternal ice sent from the heavens. Greek soldiers would rub crushed Haematite all over their bodies in preparation for battle, believing that this would make them invincible.

Whilst the ancient Greek warriors were using these minerals for protection in battle, the royal ladies of ancient Egypt, such as Cleopatra, were crushing Lapis Lazuli and Malachite to use as eye make-up, believing it would bring them physical beauty and spiritual insight. In fact, use of crystals filtered into many aspects of Egyptian life, such as the practice of placing a Quartz on the brow area of a deceased person, in preparation for their burial. This was thought to help guide the deceased gently into the after-life. Another famous example of crystal use in Egyptian times can be found in the Libyan gold tektite in Tutankhamun's scarab Wadjet pendant. The Ancient Egyptians called it 'the rock of god' and believe it invoked the power of the sun to give psychic protection to the wearer.

In some Native American traditions, crystals are referred to as the 'bones of Mother Earth' and are considered to be very powerful medicine that must be handled with love and respect. Turquoise is one stone held in the highest regard by many Native Americans. There's a beautiful myth that once upon a time after a bad drought, the Native Americans danced and wept with joy to welcome the rainfall. The rain, mixed with their tears, seeped into Mother Earth to become Turquoise. Turquoise has often been used in these indigenous cultures as jewellery and talismans, to bring protection to the wearer. If anyone ever noticed that the Turquoise they were carrying had a crack, it was understood to be a sign that the stone had protected them against some negative energies.

Science of Crystals

OK, you might be thinking, 'hang on a minute this still has woo-woo vibes all over it!' Let me give you some of the science behind crystals to help you understand the very real power of these Inner Beauty tools. Crystals are a particular form of mineral (in the same family as pebbles, pumice, marble) with a very precise pattern in their molecular structure. The molecules of a crystal are arranged in a fixed, regularly repeating geometric pattern. Because they're fixed in such a perfect way, crystals tend to remain stable over millions of years. In fact, crystals are the most ordered and stable matter in the universe and because of this they easily maintain their vibrational frequency. We know from physics that everything in the universe vibrates when observed on the molecular level. Even the ultimate brainiac Albert Einstein said, 'everything in life is a vibration.' Just because the naked human eye can't detect these vibrations doesn't mean they don't occur.

As crystals are able to maintain their vibrational frequency, they're better than any other substance in the known physical universe at transmitting energy forms in a specific direction. This is why Quartz crystal is the standard material used to ensure watches keep time, and why silicon chips (silicon is a crystal) are used in computers. We can best understand the importance of crystals and their stability if we consider how unstable the human body is, which is changing all the time. It's known that every seven years, most cells in your body are replaced. Even in our own experience, we can see how quickly physical attributes like our skin, and invisible attributes like our thoughts and feelings, change from moment to moment.

So it's really amazing that we have these beautiful objects from Mother Earth that, because they're so stable, can help us very changeable humans to do amazing things like keep time and communicate vast amounts of information via our computers.

'Crystals are better than any other substance in the known physical universe at transmitting energy forms in a specific direction.'

How Crystals Heal

Crystals are the eyes, the ears, the nose and the mouth of the Earth, which uses them to see, to hear, to smell and to taste. It is also through them that it communicates with its other brothers and sisters, with the planets in the solar system. Each crystal taken from the earth maintains its contact with the heart of the earth.

Luc Bourgault

Beauty is itself a powerful form of healing. When I'm feeling out of sorts or a little run down, I'll often go and treat myself to a bunch of sweet-smelling flowers like hyacinths, roses or freesias. I place them in my view and just let their beauty uplift me throughout the day. And crystals are, in my mind, some of the most beautiful objects in the world.

But beyond their natural beauty, crystals have been known and used for their magical healing powers for thousands of years. So how do crystals heal? Well, like so many healing tools and medicines, we're not 100 per cent sure. There are, however, some explanations that make a lot of sense to me. Remember that crystals have a consistent molecular structure which makes them really good at keeping time? When we humans are in harmony, all parts of us (thoughts, feelings, cells, organs) are working together to support each other: our inner world is like one big happy family. On one level, crystals heal because, through their highly consistent molecular structure, they bring inconsistent energies back into harmony. When you come into contact with a crystal, you become synchronized with that crystal's specific signature frequency. This bringing back into harmony is known as 'entrainment'.

To understand entrainment, I like to think about walking down a very busy street: there are car horns honking, machines drilling, people shouting, the air is full of pollution. My heart starts beating faster, and my system gets tense as it 'entrains' to this chaotic scene. On the other hand, if I go home from this scene, light some candles, play some relaxing music and create a nice bath ritual for myself, then my heart slows down and my body relaxes, as my system entrains to the different vibrations. We actually entrain to rhythms all the time, although we're usually not aware of this process. There are many examples of entrainment in nature, such as fireflies that entrain to each other so that their flashes of light happen in a perfect harmony. And it's usually the weaker, more chaotic, less stable vibration that will entrain to the stronger, more consistent, more stable vibration. This is why crystals are so amazing: because they're so consistent, their vibration so stable, we naturally entrain to them. Alongside this, crystals support our intentions. Once we have used a particular crystal in a ritual or even if we've just been sitting with it, it then serves as an energetically charged and beautiful reminder of the intention we have set.

During my time spent with Native and South American wisdom-keepers, my eyes were opened to a deeper understanding of how crystals heal us. My teachers shared with me that the stones they worked with contained the spiritual energy of the place they came from. In Andean wisdom, some of the most powerful energies or spirits are associated with the sacred mountains (*apus*). When a person is on pilgrimage around one of their sacred mountains, a stone or crystal might call out to them. This stone (*khuya*) will contain the highly charged energy of that particular mountain's spirit. This energy can then be taken with a person in the form of the stone, and that stone will be used for healing.

So, how can you incorporate the healing energies of crystals into your home and everyday life in a way that will help your Inner Beauty unfold? A good way to start is by adding a few crystals to your sacred space. Overleaf, you'll find an overview of some of the main crystals. As you continue to read through this book, you'll find different rituals that use crystals in different ways. For example, on page 131 there's a ritual related to sleep, which involves placing certain crystals in your bedroom. Another great way of connecting with the healing energy of crystals in your everyday life is wearing crystals in jewellery. I have a collection of different crystal necklaces that I choose depending on which energies I want to connect with that day. You can also carry crystals around with you in your pocket or close to your body. In the Andean tradition, people carry their crystals and stones in a special cloth along with other sacred items, and this whole bundle is called a *mesa*. (More on this on page 144.)

People often ask me, 'How do I know what is the best crystal for me?' The best advice I can give is to trust your intuition. Go with what speaks to your heart, what feels right. When you're looking at crystals you might be attracted to a specific one visually. When you hold a crystal, you might feel a certain connection. Pay close attention when holding a crystal to whether it gives you a certain positive feeling on the inside. I often think that crystals pick us rather than us picking them.

Overview of Some of the Main Crystals ▽

Rose Quartz

Rose Quartz is a beautiful pink stone belonging to the Quartz family. It's known as the stone of love and is associated with the heart, radiating calming energies of compassion and nurture. Rose Quartz is like the soft pink rose, opening its petals to reveal its heart and true beauty. In ancient Egypt, women would add powdered Rose Quartz to their beauty creams, believing it would bring them eternal beauty and youthfulness. Later in this book, I'll share some beauty tips with you that include Rose Quartz to spice up your normal beauty routine. I love what Joy Gardner says of Rose Quartz, 'For those who have been hurt in love, Rose Quartz is the Divine Mother who rocks you in her arms whilst she exudes unconditional love.'

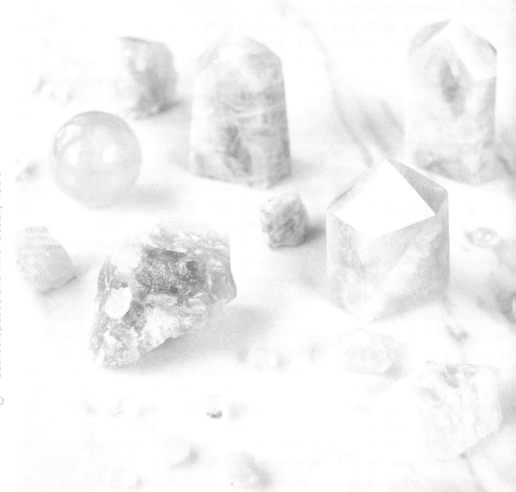

Amethyst

Amethyst reflects peaceful tones of light to deep purple. This crystal is known to bring inner peace and protection. Luc Bourgault, who wrote one of my favourite books on crystals *The American Indian Secrets of Crystal Healing*, shares his thoughts on Amethyst as a powerful protector stone: 'Amethyst is the stone of travel … a number of people have told me that the Amethyst in their car has saved their lives.' The word 'Amethyst' originates from the Greek word meaning 'sober'. The Ancient Greeks believed that goblets carved from Amethyst would help protect them and ensure they remained sober whilst drinking their wine. I can't say I've tried this one myself, but I do love the idea of Amethyst cups! Amethyst is a wonderful tool to use during meditation and spiritual work. The dreamy purple shades of the stone evoke a sense of calmness, like the fragrance of crushed lavender in the palm of your hand. Because of this calming and peaceful quality, Amethyst is also a perfect crystal to place on your night-stand, helping to promote a peaceful and relaxing energy for a good night's sleep. In fact, it was believed in biblical times that this stone could induce powerful dreams and visions. I personally always have a piece of Amethyst on my night-stand. Whenever I cast my eyes on it, I feel a sense of protection and calm before I drift off.

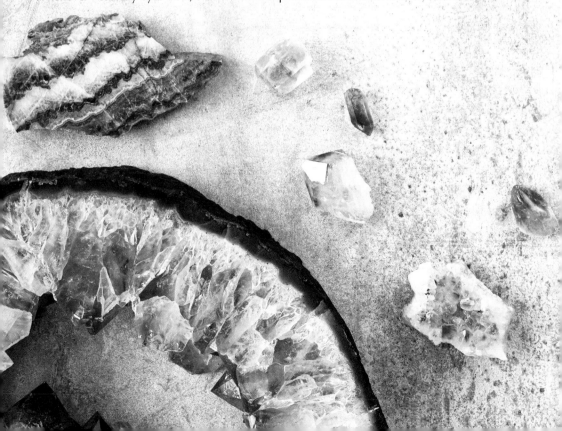

Clear Quartz

Clear Quartz is known as one of the master crystals of the mineral kingdom. This crystal has a beautiful colourless transparency. So you can understand why the ancient Greeks believed it to be eternal ice sent from the Gods. Clear Quartz is associated with the Crown Chakra and helps to bring the energies of focus and clarity, which can be a great companion whenever you're in need of wise decision making. Clear Quartz is also a powerful amplifier of energy, making it a wonderful crystal to help boost vitality. I often carry a piece of Clear Quartz with me to meetings to help me stay focussed, energized and on the ball.

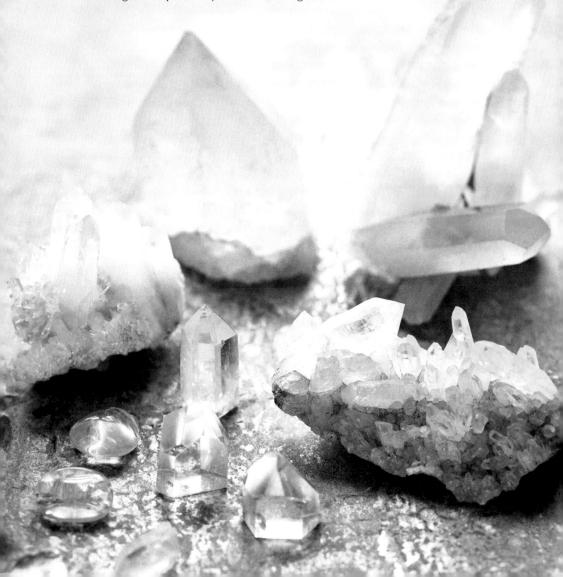

Moonstone

Moonstone comes from the Feldspar family of minerals. In ancient times in Mother India, Moonstone was a popular wedding gift. It was also believed that placing Moonstone in the mouth of a lover during the full moon would bestow blessings on the couple's future together. Moonstone really embodies the feminine energy, the inner goddess. I particularly love Rainbow Moonstone as it has these amazing iridescent flashes that reflect the colours of the rainbow. This stone is a perfect example of the natural beauty of Mother Earth. Seeing this stone reflect the different colours of the rainbow is like a mirror to the different tones of our own Inner Beauty qualities. I personally love to use Moonstone when I want to tap into my feminine energy: powerful but serene.

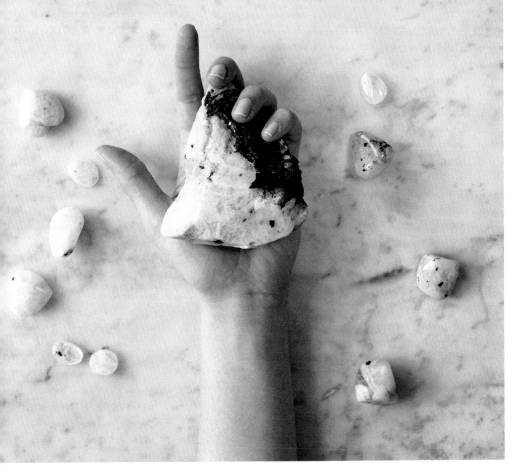

Citrine

Citrine is part of the Quartz family and is named after the French word for lemon (*citron*). Because of its iron inclusion and other geological effects, it reflects the colour yellow, ranging from soft yellows to brown. Citrine is like the sun, shining its illuminating rays through the grey skies down on to the Earth, helping to uplift and energize everything that is touched by its light. This stone is also wonderful to manifest abundance and prosperity. As Naisha Ahsian says in *The Book of Stones*: 'When one chooses the path of love and joy, opening to the power of divine will, Citrine supports us in bringing forth what is truly beautiful.' A common variety of Citrine that is readily available is actually Amethyst or Smoky Quartz that has been heat-treated to make Citrine, emulating how Citrine is naturally formed in Mother Earth. Heat-treated Citrine tends to be a brighter orange/yellow colour, whilst natural Citrine often appears as a light, soft yellow or browner tone. Many people feel heat-treated Citrine still has the healing properties of natural Citrine. I like both, but I sense that natural Citrine is more potent. I recommend you try working with one or the other and see whether it resonates with you.

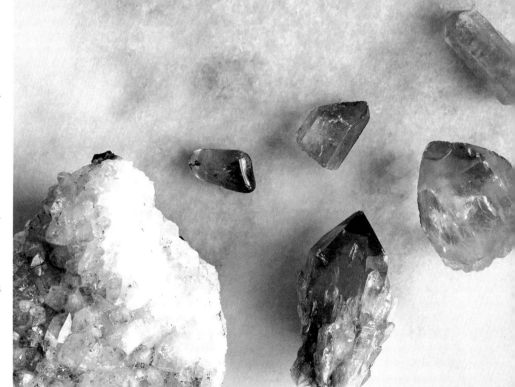

Fluorite

Fluorite comes in a wonderful rainbow of colours. It's a really good stone to help brainstorm creative projects, to bring these creative ideas into form, and to weave a thread of beauty throughout. For this reason I love to place Rainbow Fluorite on my work desk. When I look at the layers of colour and pattern in this stone, I feel inspired by Nature's own creativity.

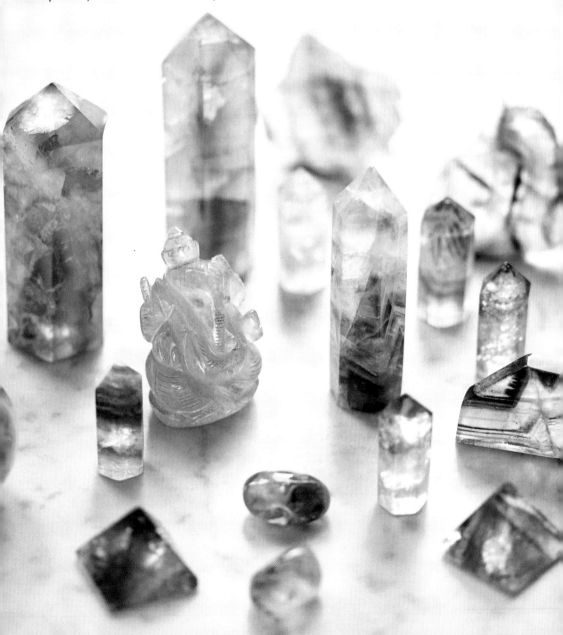

Lapis Lazuli

Lapis Lazuli is a beautiful deep-blue stone made from a mix of minerals including Sodalite, flecks of Pyrite, and streaks of white Calcite. Because of its royal blue colouring it's associated with the Third Eye. It helps to bring spiritual insight, making Lapis a wonderful stone to use for deep meditation, especially when we want a deeper understanding of a situation. In Mahayana Buddhism, the name for the 'Medicine Buddha' – the Buddha who cures suffering through the medicine of his wisdom teaching – is translated as 'King of Medicine Master and Lapis Lazuli Light'. One of the twelve sacred vows read in worship of this Buddha reads: 'To awaken the minds of sentient beings through his light of Lapis Lazuli.' I find this ancient vision very powerful and true, and often find great healing through insight when working with this stone. The Royal Egyptians also celebrated the special energy of Lapis, crushing it and using it as eyeliner, but also adorning their necks with Lapis stones to bring them insight and truth.

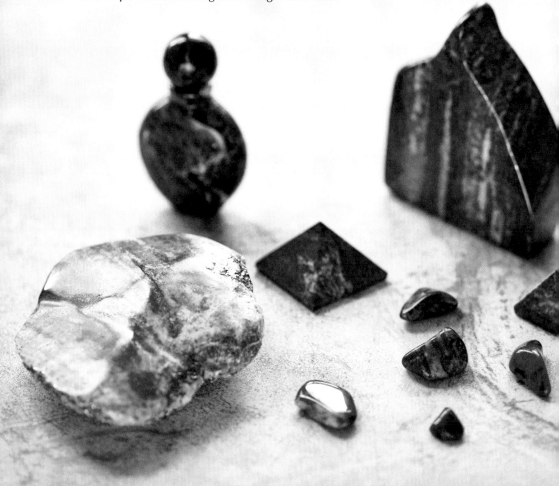

Turquoise

Turquoise is a beautiful, opaque, blue to green stone. It's used to bring protection and to help us connect to ancient spiritual wisdom. The beauty of Turquoise has been highly praised by many cultures and is a popular choice for a talisman (a talisman is basically an object that brings luck and protection). The Navajo people regard Turquoise as one of their most sacred stones, using it for special ceremonies and offerings. Overall, Turquoise is a wonderful tool to wear in jewellery because it not only looks beautiful, but it also brings protection, especially when travelling. The stone supports shamanic journeying, which for me means gaining access to other profound dimensions of our experience. I personally love using Turquoise when I want to go deep in my meditation and connect back to lessons learned from wisdom-keepers I've met.

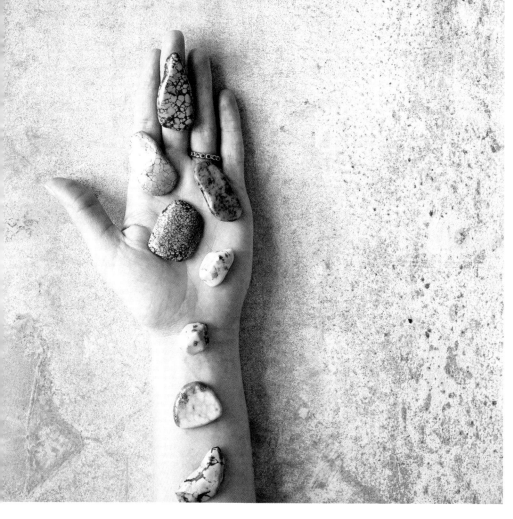

Cleansing Crystals

Crystals can hold unwanted, heavy or old energy, so it's important to cleanse them regularly. Cleansing is especially important when you acquire a new crystal, or when you've been using a particular crystal a lot, especially through a difficult situation. Cleansing a crystal allows the true healing powers and beauty of the stone to shine. There are many ways of cleansing from the simpler, more practical methods to more elaborate techniques that weave a deeper sense of ritual into the process. I have my own favourite ways of cleansing which I'll share with you now, but I recommend you always go for the way that intuitively works best for your own self.

One of the simplest but most graceful ways of purifying a crystal is through smudging tools such as sage or Palo Santo wood. These tools, when burned, produce a distinctive smell and smoke. When I burn them, I move the tool slowly, mindfully, around the crystal, watching the smoke dance a cleansing trail, lifting unwanted energies and carrying them off and away. I always have a window open whenever possible, as this gives the unwanted energies an escape route. We'll look in more detail at specific smudging tools on page 60.

If you have quite a few crystals to cleanse in one go, the most practical and quickest way to do this is through sound. Striking a singing bowl a couple of times, or sounding chimes (*tingsha*), over your crystals will very quickly help to bring your stones back to their most harmonious state.

If you like the idea of using a water-based cleansing ritual (we clean ourselves with water after all), then you can simply run your crystals under some pure water. Natural running water is best here, but running the crystals under your cold tap will do too, as the flow of the water will drain away the unwanted energies. Just a heads-up: some crystals are not water-friendly due to their toxicity or softness, so please check with a complete toxic crystal list for this.

If you're lucky enough to live near clear, natural water, then I really recommend you take your crystals there to cleanse every once in a while. There is really no more poetic place to cleanse your crystals than the pure, flowing waters of a stream, river or sea. There's a Zen saying I just love: 'Be like a rock in the middle of a river, let all of the water flow around and past you.' As I live in the city of London, sadly I don't have any such clean water near me. But, whenever I go out of London, I like to bring my crystals with me. Recently, on a break in the stunning

Cotswold countryside with my husband, we went for a walk and found a beautiful stream at the source of the River Thames. The energy was so peaceful there. As I stood by the side of the stream, I said a small blessing and carefully held my crystals one by one in the flowing water, allowing Mother Nature to cleanse their energy (make sure you have a good grasp of the crystal as you don't want it to float away!). Always give thanks to the spirit of the water. You might also like to collect some of the water in an empty bottle, so you can take it home and use it at a later date.

When I want to give my crystals a really deep cleanse, I bury them in the earth. I particularly choose this cleansing method when I've received a new crystal or if I've been using a particular crystal a lot. This method really helps to direct any old or unwanted energies away from the crystal and back into the earth. You can make this process into more of a ritual by saying a small blessing before burying it into the earth. In this cleansing ritual, I give thanks to the crystal for the support it has and will continue to give me, and then I offer the energies back into the earth. In Andean spirituality, Pachamama loves nothing more than to absorb our heavy energies (*hucha*). Our heavy energy is like food for her, which she effortlessly digests and converts into sweet, refined energy (*sami*). I normally leave the crystal buried in the earth for at least a full day and night, often for a couple of days and sometimes even a week, depending on the level of cleansing that I feel is needed for particular crystals.

I appreciate this might not be accessible to everyone, especially living in the city, where many of us don't even have a garden. In that case, you could bury your crystals in a big bowl of sand or the soil of a plant and leave this bowl or plant on your balcony or somewhere it won't get knocked over.

The last (but definitely not the least) method that I'll share with you involves bathing the crystals under the moonlight. The moon has such a very powerful and beautiful energy. In many cultures, it has been just as important to honour the cycles of the moon as it has been to honour the sun. So with this in mind, place your crystals outside in your garden, or on your window-ledge for an evening, and simply let the beautiful rays of the moon cleanse the energy of your stones. I try to do this monthly under the full moon, along with a meditation or saying a small blessing over the crystals, before leaving them to cleanse under the moonlight. It does not need to be a full moon, but obviously full moons are more potent (as you will see in the Nature Rituals section, page 152 onwards).

SMUDGING/CLEANSING TOOLS

You know when you've just had one of those days, those days when the universe seems to be really testing you; maybe there have been some awkward conversations, an unfriendly glare from a stranger, an argument with a colleague, friend or partner. And when you come home you notice still lingering somewhere in your body that uncomfortable residual energy. I know when I've had one of those days the first thing I like to do is have a long hot shower or a bath. As soon as the hot water hits my body, I can really begin to feel lighter emotionally, as the tension washes away down the plug hole. This very same idea of cleansing away heavy energies lies behind the ancient practices of smudging or cleansing rituals. With these rituals, you're using sound, smell and smoke to cleanse these energies. Oh, and these practices are great because you can use them anywhere: at home, in the office, on the move. You can smudge yourself, you can smudge objects (like crystals), and you can smudge spaces. It's an all-round key ingredient for Inner Beauty.

Smudging specifically refers to the burning of certain herbs or woods, creating a sacred smoke. The smoke, combined with intention, helps to get rid of any stagnant or heavy energies. This practice has been used by Native Americans and many other traditional cultures for a long time.

There are many different smudging tools including sage, sweet grass, cedar wood, sandalwood, but my number one favourite is the sacred wood of the Palo Santo tree. The name Palo Santo means 'holy wood', and these wooden sticks, taken directly from the sacred tree in South America, give off a heavenly minty, citrus scent when burned. I'm such a sucker for things that smell so heavenly! The wood has been used in ritual and ceremony since the time of the Inca civilization to ward off *mala* (bad) energy. In Peru, many of the shops have bowls filled with burning Palo Santo wood, so that the smoke cleanses customers as they enter.

These sticks are so easy to use. I simply light one end until the wood is burning and there is enough smoke being generated, then I let the smoke trail around the area or object I want to cleanse. It can really help to have a large shell – abalone shells are ideal – to collect the ash and embers whilst you burn your smudging tool of choice.

In the Native American way, herbs such as sage are bundled together and burned, and the sacred smoke that arises is believed to carry the prayers and blessings of the person doing the smudging up to the heavens. White sage is a great tool

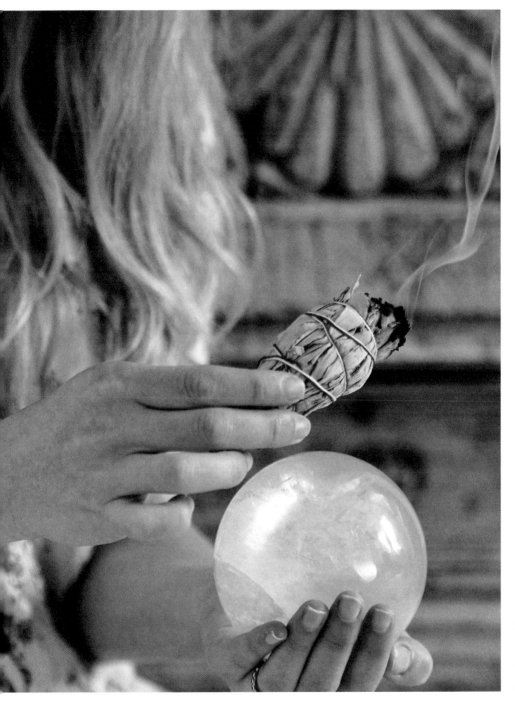

Sacred Spaces and Inner Beauty Tools

to use when you've moved into a new house or office space as it creates a lot of smoke, and so allows you to move through a space, and give it a real deep, energetic cleanse. Traditionally, a feather is used to waft over the ignited end to help maintain the smoke but also to welcome in the spirit of air. An interesting, modern variation on smudging practice that I learned from a Chumash wisdom-keeper and friend is to use sage to cleanse any second-hand or vintage clothes or other used items you may acquire before using them. Although I like the smell of sage, I do find it can be a bit overwhelming sometimes, so I like to add a small amount of dried lavender which helps to sweeten the aroma as well as bringing a calming energy. It's always important when smudging to make sure there's a way for the smoke to carry unwanted energies outside; so make sure there is at least one window open, if possible.

Another great way to cleanse the energy of your space is by creating crystal-infused spritzers. I particularly love using this method as it's super-quick, but also because crystals are involved! So, first thing you'll need is a small glass bottle with a spritzer top. If you don't have one at home already, you can easily find these online. The next step is to choose your crystals. Some of my favourites for cleansing are Snowy Quartz or Amethyst. Ideally, you want to use very small, polished tumble stones or small polished crystal chips. Always make sure the crystals you're using have been cleansed and that you've placed your own blessing or intention on to them. Next, place the crystals in the bottle and fill it with filtered or natural mineral water. To intensify the potency of the cleanse and to add a lovely smell, put a couple of drops of essential oil into the spritzer. Some oils I might add that are also associated with cleansing are either lemon oil, peppermint, holy basil or Palo Santo oil. Now you have your spritzer ready, you can go spritz away, making the energy of your home all fresh, sparkly and clean.

'Another great way to cleanse the energy of your space is by creating crystal-infused spritzers.'

NATURAL OBJECTS

'In Nature, nothing is perfect and everything is perfect. Trees can be contorted, bent in weird ways, and they're still beautiful.'
Alice Walker

I often think that we're so lucky to have been born here on Mother Earth, surrounded by so much beauty in Nature. It's as though Nature is constantly giving us little clues about the beauty inside ourselves. We are after all a part of Nature, not separate from it, and I find it's helpful to remember this every now and then. Even when natural things are old and decaying, I still appreciate them, sometimes even more so. Have you ever looked in awe at a big old tree that has really magical, twisting roots and branches? Ram Dass, one of my favourite teachers, describes the power of Nature so well: 'When you go out into the woods and you look at trees, you see all these different trees. And some of them are bent, and some of them are straight, and some of them are evergreens, and some of them are whatever. And you look at the tree and you allow it. You appreciate it. You see why it is the way it is. You sort of understand that it didn't get enough light, and so it turned that way. And you don't get all emotional about it. You just allow it. You appreciate the tree.'

So you can probably get why I love using natural objects as ingredients for Inner Beauty rituals. Before we look at specific kinds of natural objects, it's important to remember that, when we're taking objects from nature, we always need to do so in a way that is respectful and appreciative. I much prefer to use things I've found, e.g. that have fallen from a tree, or drifted on to a beach. If you want to take something from a plant or flower, a nice way to do it is to check in with yourself to see if it feels right to take that object; you can even ask the plant or flower for permission, and then always give thanks to Nature for providing these beautiful tools.

Before you read on, take a minute to reflect: what's a favourite memory for you of being in Nature? Where were you: in the woods, on the beach, in a field? What could you smell, see, hear? What did you feel inside? Let these feelings be your guide as you choose objects to connect to your own deeper, beautiful Nature.

Trees

'Keep a green tree in your heart and perhaps a singing bird will come.'
Chinese proverb

I like to think of trees as the most sturdy and reliable of friends. Trees are so resilient and have such rugged beauty that I always take time to appreciate them whenever I'm walking in Nature. With roots so connected to the earth and branches reaching out to heaven, trees can help us both to stay grounded and to dream. And we have a vital connection with trees. As Les Stroud says: 'When we exhale, a tree breathes in. When a tree exhales, we breathe in.' One of my most joyful memories was getting married in a beautiful woodland glade, surrounded by slender, tall Birch trees (I loved finding out recently that Birch trees are known as the Goddess Trees or 'The Lady of the Woods'). Did you know that trees actually communicate and support each other through their own kind of internet: complex underground networks of fungi that connect them to each other?

Trees have unsurprisingly been celebrated for their wisdom throughout the ages. In India for example, the fig tree is particularly sacred and is believed to represent the human psyche and to be a dwelling place for the gods. You may already know that the Buddha was said to have attained enlightenment whilst sitting under the Bodhi tree, which was a very old and sacred fig tree. Do you have any special memories associated with trees?

My favourite Inner Beauty tool I borrow from the tree world is simply driftwood. Although I don't live near a beach, whenever I get a chance, I love to visit the seaside and look for unusual, beautiful pieces of driftwood to add to my sacred space. There's something about the mysterious journey that driftwood has taken to arrive at this point that gives these pieces a magical quality.

Pine cones are also wonderful additions to your Inner Beauty kit. Pine trees are seen in folklore as homes for fairies, as well as being welcoming, refreshing places where tired travellers could catch a moment's rest in the protective space of the tree. Pine cones are known to carry this protective energy, and so they can be placed anywhere in your home or office environment to create that fresh sense of rejuvenation and support. Pine cones are also wonderful to use to decorate your sacred space in autumn, along with those beautiful purple, russet red and orange leaves, oak sprigs and acorns.

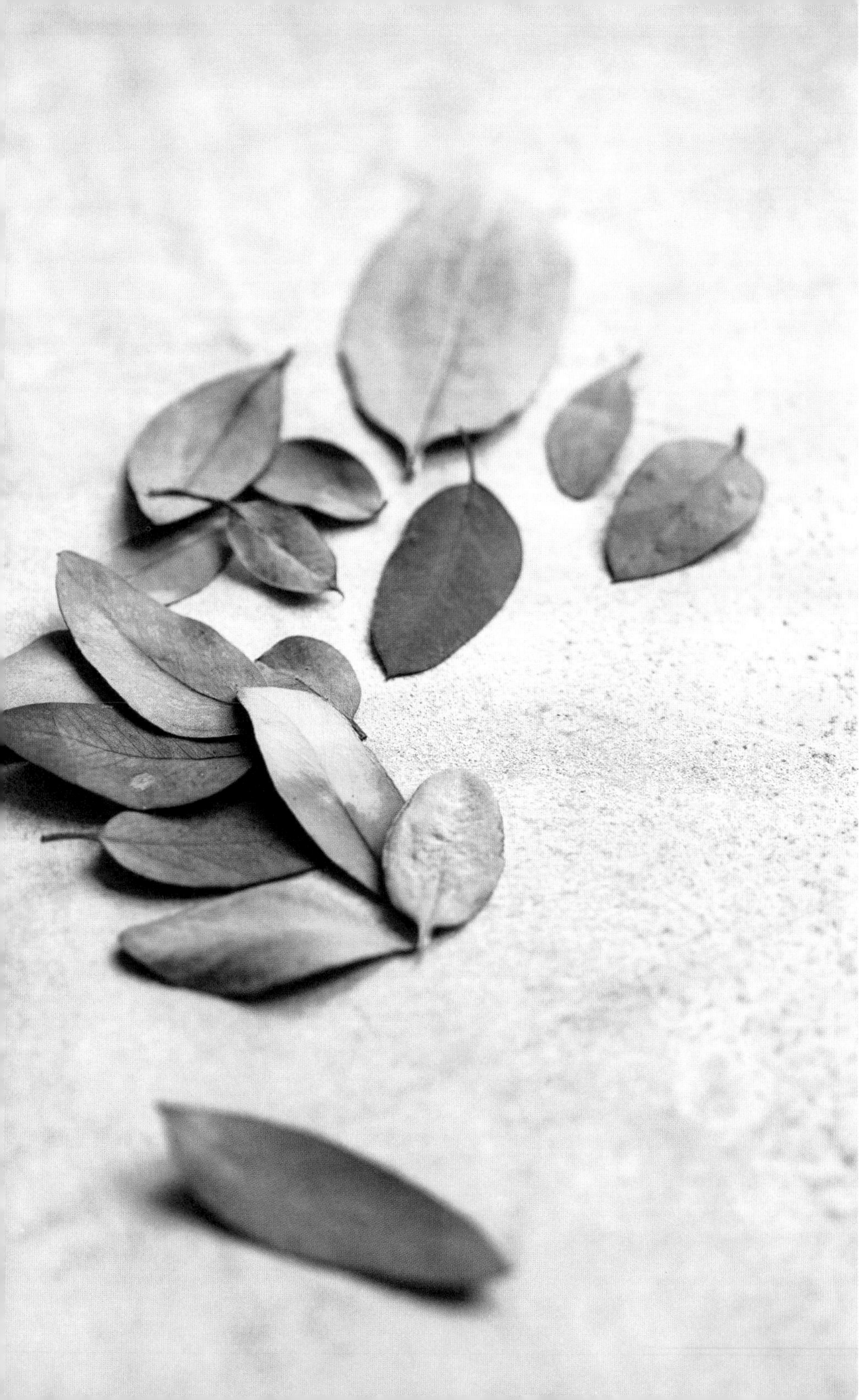

Flowers

'Earth laughs in flowers.'
    Ralph Waldo Emerson

Flowers bring vibrant colour and beauty to any space. There are few places where flowers aren't welcome. Flowers are sacred affirmations in the cycle of life, used to mark all the major transitions of a human life, from birth, to celebration, to death. How do you bring flowers into your world?

I really recommend not waiting for the next birthday or special event to bring more flowers into your life. Flowers will brighten up your every day, bringing warm love and life into your heart, through your eyes and your nose. And there is a much deeper dimension to these pretty, fragrant friends. Flowers have healing energies. For example, both Tibetan Buddhists and the Shipibo tribes from the Amazonian basin of Peru use flower-infused water to bathe people. These 'flower baths' are said to cleanse heavy energies and to restore balance. Doesn't this just sound dreamy? When I spent some time in Peru, I took part in ceremonies (*despachos*) where the grandmother wisdom-keeper would collect the most beautiful flowers, adding them to the sacred offerings in beautiful mandala-like creations. For an example of flowers' healing power in more modern times, just consider how many people like a nice cup of camomile tea to relax themselves.

Almost any flower can add vitality, beauty and joy to a sacred space, but there are some flowers that are more powerful healing agents, and which are wisely used in Inner Beauty rituals. My favourites are scented flowers such as hyacinths, lavender, and of course roses. Hyacinths have the most stunning smell, and so it's no surprise that their perfume has been celebrated for thousands of years for helping us let go of the past and to find focus in the present. In Ancient Egypt, hyacinths were used to help people grieve. I love to add hyacinths to my sacred space, especially when I'm feeling a little low and want to let go of some old memories. I'm sure you know that lavender is a very calming and sleep-inducing flower. Medicinally, lavender oil can also help to relieve stress, to heal burns and bites, and as a mood-booster. Even in Roman times, lavender was used in sacred bathing rituals. I personally use lavender as an Inner Beauty ingredient whenever I'm feeling stressed and need to reconnect to that peaceful place within. I love to crush lavender in my hands and just breathe in the aroma that is released. Roses,

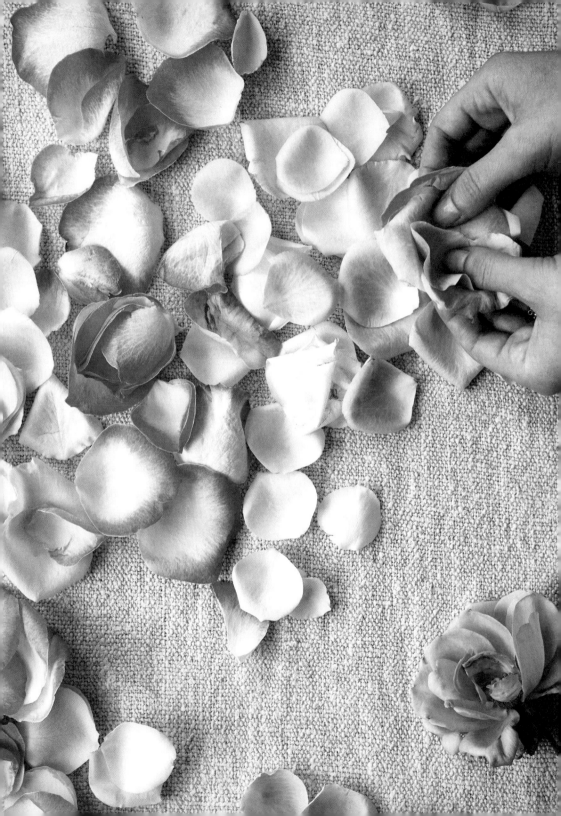

as you already know, have been a love of mine since childhood. I fell in love with roses even more when my husband proposed to me in a rose garden overlooking the Old City of Jerusalem. And then, on my honeymoon, whilst travelling around India, I discovered the most deliciously fragrant roses. This was in the holy town of Pushkar in Rajasthan, where the town is literally surrounded on all sides by these beautiful wild rose fields. It's also one of my favourite ingredients in beauty products, especially skincare. Along with a smell that never fails to send my heart fluttering, rose is moisturizing, toning and anti-ageing. And, as an Inner Beauty tool, rose is of course the classic symbol of Love. In Sufi poetic wisdom, the beauty of the rose is what brings the nightingale to sing. Listen to these gorgeous words from the Sufi poet Hafiz:

> How
> Did the rose
> Ever open its heart
>
> And give to this world
> All its Beauty?
>
> It felt the encouragement of light
>
> Against its Being,
>
> Otherwise,
> We all remain
>
> Too Frightened.

I love using roses in my sacred space and rituals as they remind me of the Inner Beauty we all have within, that just needs the right light to reveal itself in all its glory.

Ask yourself now if there are certain flowers you feel particularly drawn to. Whenever you go for a walk in Nature, get to know the flowers that are growing around you. Feel them. Touch them. Smell them. Nature is calling to your Inner Beauty through flowers, if you let her in.

Feathers

Feathers are wonderful, multi-dimensional Inner Beauty tools that have been used in sacred and magical ways throughout human history. They are often believed to represent the heavens and celestial wisdom, and so using a feather in rituals would often be seen as a symbol of divine knowledge. Feathers also symbolize lightness and the air element. Depending on where you live, you can often find beautiful feathers just by walking around. Particular feathers that you may want to use as one of your Inner Beauty tools include: crow feathers, which represent the inner world; swan feathers, which represent grace and balance; swallow feathers, which represent light, purity, birth; and owl feathers, which represent wisdom. I always have feathers in my sacred space, and love to use feathers in certain rituals, especially rituals involving cleansing. When you are burning smudging herbs, you can use a feather to waft the smoke around a space or a person.

'Feathers are often believed to represent the heavens and celestial wisdom, and so using a feather in rituals would often be seen as a symbol of divine knowledge.'

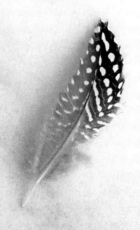

Shells

Shells provide a calming, gentle, nurturing connection to the spirit of water. We've already seen how shells were used in the oldest burial rituals. They've also been used as symbols of female fertility, as representatives of the god Vishnu in Hinduism, as healing objects to restore spirit to mind and body in Hawaiian tradition, and even as tools to divine the future in ancient Caribbean spirituality. In Native American tradition, the Abalone shell (which is a particularly beautiful shell) is used to hold burning sage as part of a smudging ritual. I personally love having seashells in the sacred spaces around my house, as they bring me back to my childhood and sweet memories of walks along the beach in search of the prettiest specimens, and occasionally holding them to my ear to hear the sea. I find seashells work really well to bring that flowing energy of the ocean into ritual.

If you live near to or ever go on a trip to the seaside, I really recommend taking some time to go searching for your very own sacred shells. This is one of my favourite things to do; it's an amazing meditation, especially with children, and I'll often bring back a bag full of beautiful shells that I'll place around the house, and use in my Inner Beauty rituals.

Stones

In the Peruvian tradition we studied, it's not just crystals that are the sacred objects from the mineral family. Stones (*khuyas*) found in sacred or special places, such as mountains, forests, by bodies of water, all contain the energy of that special place. The word *khuya* in Quechua means 'affection' or 'love', and these power stones can hold a person's desire to give kindness and love to the world. So, whenever you are out in Nature, keep your eyes peeled for any stones or pebbles that call out to you. I personally love finding stones with holes in, as I will pass strong thread through them and hang them up as a beautiful, sacred decoration.

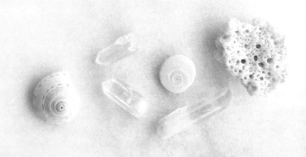

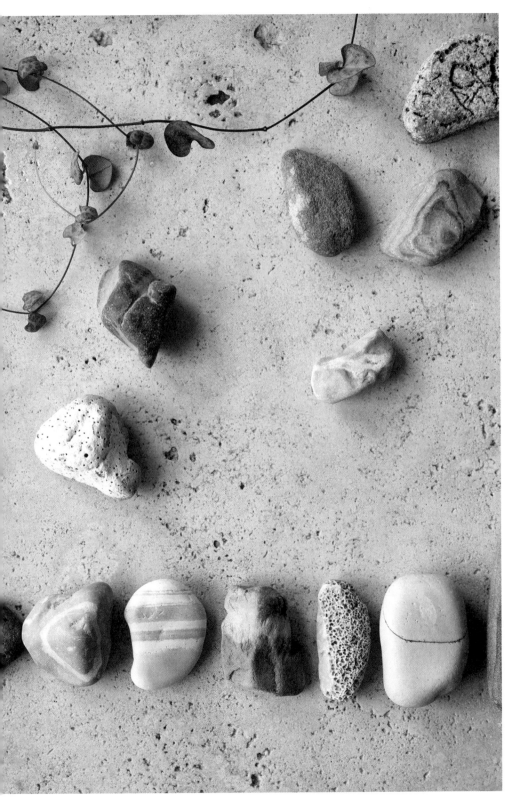

Sacred Spaces and Inner Beauty Tools

Essential Oils and Other Smells

'Perfumes are the feelings of flowers.'
    Heinrich Heine

Essential oils are poetry for the nose. I often think of each of my different essential oils as being like a key that I choose to unlock different qualities in my inner world. And these oils have been used for healing purposes since ancient times. As children, we learned of the Three Wise Kings bringing gifts of Gold, Frankincense and Myrrh to the baby Jesus. I remember thinking at the time, what would a baby do with these gifts? Well, some scholars suggest it may have been simply to evoke healing … it seems these kings were called 'wise' for a reason!

Frankincense is one of my favourite essential oils. The sacred, woody smell somehow makes me feel connected to ancient spiritual wisdom. I like to burn Frankincense to relax and enhance my meditations. My preference is for Frankincense from the *Boswellia sacra* tree, as it's 100 per cent pure and well known for its healing qualities. I often just place a couple of drops in the palm of my hand and breathe the fragrance in. I find this really helps to lift my mood. Frankincense has actually been used for medicinal purposes for thousands of years, as it was thought to be a fantastic anti-inflammatory, as well as treating many other ailments. So, this one is an all-round winner!

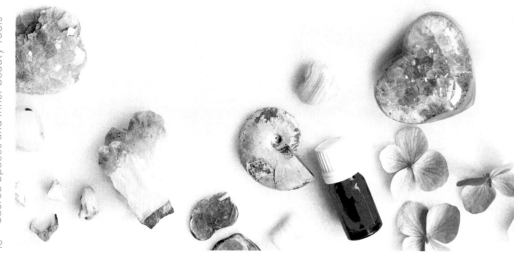

Another favourite oil of mine is of course rose oil. Rose oil comes in two main types, Rose Absolute and Rose Otto. I find Rose Absolute has a more delicate, sweet fragrance. Rose Otto has a stronger and spicier fragrance. It's really a personal choice though, so try them out for yourself and see which you prefer. Overall, I find the fragrance of rose oil very calming, nurturing and heart-centring. I absolutely love the romantic tale of the origins of rose oil. It is said that an Ottoman Emperor once ordered the fountains and canals in the royal gardens to be filled with roses to celebrate his wedding to his princess. When later walking through the gardens with her husband, the Princess noticed that an oily residue had collected on the surface of the water. She ran her fingers through the scented water and was delighted to find that a fragrant oil clung to her hands. From then on, the Emperor had it produced and bottled as a tribute to her. How romantic is that?

Like the flower that it's derived from, rose oil is known to have many wonderful healing properties. Above all, it's an amazing tool to bring peace and balance. I like to use rose oil when I'm feeling anxious, particularly if I've got a big job on the next day with a new client. I'll put some into my diffuser and allow my mind and body to just bathe in the healing fragrance. I sometimes even carry a bottle around with me, so that when I'm having a super-busy day, I can just whip it out, hold the bottle under my nose and instantly reconnect to my inner garden. Interestingly, the calming effect of rose oil was scientifically proven in 2009 in an amazing study where one group had rose oil applied to their skin, and the other had a placebo oil.[3] Amazingly, the rose oil produced a much greater relaxation response (slower breathing and even lower blood pressure) than that of the placebo oil.

Essential oils can also be used as cleansing tools. I love using Holy Basil oil (also known as Tulsi oil) to cleanse the energy of my home. This oil has a warm and spicy aroma that instantly transports me to an olde-worlde land full of magical spices and herbs. It is from an Indian plant that is purposefully grown around sacred places to help protect them from negative energy. The oil is used extensively in Indian Ayurvedic practice to help relieve stress and to support the immune system. I love to add a couple of drops to a tissue and breathe in the aroma before I begin my morning meditations. I find it really helps to clear my head. When I breathe in the aromatic aroma I can feel the mind chatter soften and a sense of balance is restored.

There are of course so many other wonderful smells that you can and probably already do use as an Inner Beauty ingredient. My wish is that you get even more inspiration from reading this to pamper your nose as much as I love to! To really strengthen your connection to the amazing Inner Beauty power of sacred smells, ask yourself these questions: which smells in your life instantly relax you? Are there any smells which bring on certain moods in you (think freshly cut grass, sea air, the invigorating smell of pine trees in a forest, etc)? Which scents can you call upon as your own Inner Beauty guides?

Please note that wherever I've suggested oils in rituals, it might not be OK to put the oil neat on to the skin, especially during certain stages of pregnancy. You also may need to mix it with a carrier oil, such as almond or grapeseed oil.

'Essential oils are poetry for the nose. I often think of each of my different essential oils as being like a key that I choose to unlock different qualities in my inner world.'

Sounds

Whenever I'm feeling a bit out of sorts or disconnected from my Inner Beauty, I love playing a song like 'California' by Joni Mitchell or 'Scarborough Fair' by Simon and Garfunkel. There's something about the ethereal melodies of these songs that lifts my soul every time. I've discovered over the last few years that it's possible to conjure up the dreamy feeling of such songs in Inner Beauty rituals by using certain sacred sound instruments. Here are some of my favourite Inner Beauty instruments.

The singing bowl is the ultimate tool for centring our minds. I often think of the sound of singing bowls as being like the subtle sounds of Nature, like a bird singing or the rustle of leaves underfoot; those sounds that can bring your attention effortlessly back to one point. These instruments are called singing bowls because, as you run the striker around the edges, they start to 'sing'. When one of these bowls is holding water and made to sing, water inside the bowl literally starts to dance around the edges. I find just playing these sacred instruments is a strong heart-connecting meditation in itself. These beautiful bowls have been used traditionally, particularly in Buddhist tradition, as spiritual tools to lead people into and out of meditation. I have a few different singing bowls at home, but my favourites are Tibetan singing bowls and crystal singing bowls. In Tibetan tradition, singing bowls are said to date back to the time of the Buddha. These bowls are usually made of a number of different metals, and they make a variety of tones depending on their size. Crystal singing bowls are usually made from Quartz crystal, and they come in different sizes, each one loosely relating to a different chakra. These bowls not only make an amazing, powerful sound that is relaxing and centring, but they also carry the energy of the Quartz crystal which just amplifies their healing capacity. I particularly love putting crushed lavender or rose petals in my singing bowl, and playing the sound, and then breathing in the smell, which always seems so wonderfully enhanced.

Another favourite sound instrument of mine is the *Tingsha*, Tibetan meditation cymbals. The sound these cymbals make is much higher and more direct, and you have to play them very sensitively as otherwise it can be quite overwhelming. Again, these are amazing tools to quickly centre your mind, and they are also a perfect tool for cleansing a number of crystals in one go. My husband often recommends these to parents in his therapy practice, as there is a really fun game you can play when things are getting a bit chaotic in the house: everyone apart from the one playing the instrument closes their eyes, the cymbals are sounded, and whoever puts their hand up closest to when the sound has ended has won the game. This game seems to really help kids to slow down and tune in to their senses. In Tibetan tradition, the *Tingsha* are used in different rituals, like the Hungry Ghost ritual. In the Hungry Ghost ritual, the cymbals are played and the sound is used as an offering of compassion, to help bring liberation to the 'Hungry Ghosts' who suffer with endless desires that can never be satisfied.

Are there certain sounds that transport you to somewhere magical, or bring you instantly back to your heart and the present moment? Maybe you have a go-to song that you listen to when you need some TLC or a pick-me-up?

One of the loveliest things about the kind of sacred sounds described above is that they can help you to tune in to the silence within. In modern life, I find my mind gets so overwhelmed with noise and information. It's so important for my wellbeing that I find a way to regularly connect with silence. And these sacred sound instruments really help. When we tune into one very pure, sacred sound suddenly we become aware of the great silence that holds everything together.

So start to pay a little more attention, not only to the sounds in your environment, but also to the gaps between the sounds. Appreciate the silence as much as the noise. Many traditional and non-Western cultures have long placed a high value on silence. In indigenous Fijian communities, *vakonomodi*, or deep silence, is the greatest mark of respect one can pay to the land and to other people. Listen to this glorious description of silence from a Lakota Native American community:

'We Indians know about silence. We aren't afraid of it.
In fact, to us it is more powerful than words. Our elders
were schooled in the ways of silence, and they passed
that along to us. Watch, listen, and then act, they told us …
Watch the animals to see how they care for their young.
Watch the elders to see how they behave … Always watch
first, with a still heart and mind, then you will learn.
When you have watched enough, then you can act.'

Kent Nerburn, *Neither Wolf Nor Dog*

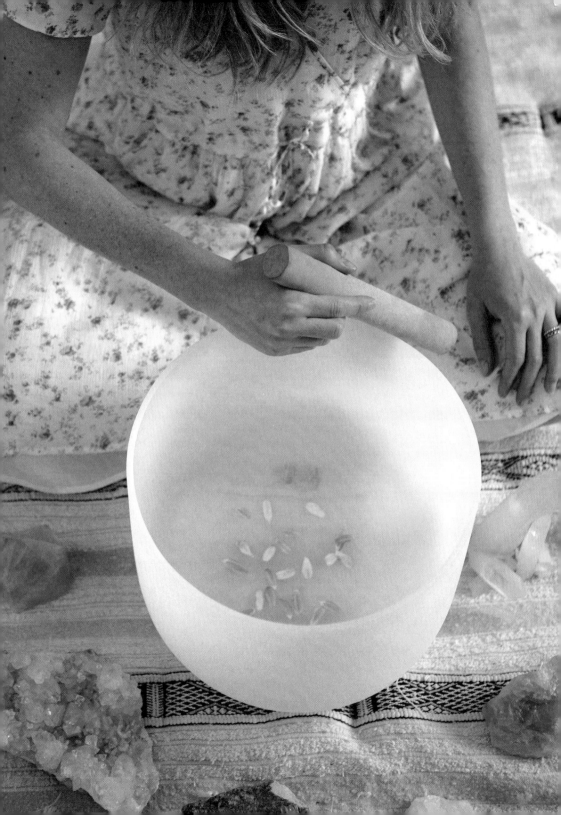

Introduction
to Rituals

3

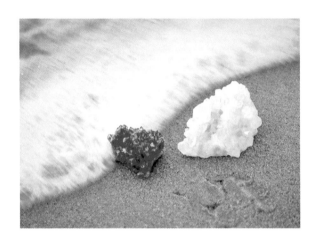
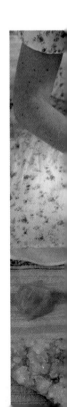

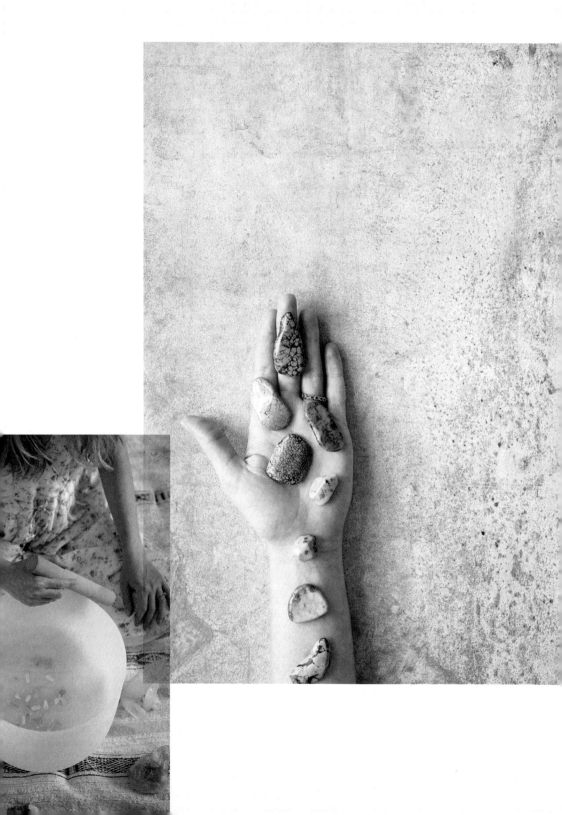

Here are some tips that will help you to get the most out of the rituals shared in the following sections.

Start Small but Do Something

♥

There are lots of different suggestions in this book for what Inner Beauty tools to use and how to use them in ritual. But the most important thing is consistency. It's better to start with small steps that you can keep up, and then build on, rather than trying to begin with everything all at once and then feeling like a failure when you forget or lose track. I've tried to base some of the rituals in this book on things that you might already do. This is called habit stacking, and it makes it much easier to add a little magic to your routine. So if this world of rituals is completely new to you, don't get overwhelmed. Choose small simple steps to start with, and you can build from there. But get inspired and do something! The magic of ritual awaits your action.

Importance of Time and Space

♥

When doing a ritual, we want to create a space where magic can happen. If you do your ritual in the same rushed way as you might plough through your emails or hurry through the washing up, it's unlikely the ritual will have the desired effect. So, even as you are preparing the space for the ritual, try to allow your mind to settle down, tune in to your senses as you gather your Inner Beauty tools, allow every movement, every gesture, every word to be deliberate and filled with a loving intention. When we are doing a ritual, we ideally want to create that magical feeling that we are stepping into another world, a world different from our everyday reality. Make sure that you can be free from distraction for as long as the ritual takes.

Cleanse

♥

It's important to cleanse at the start of every ritual. We want to make sure that the space, the Inner Beauty tools and ourselves are free from any stagnant, heavy or unwanted energy before we start the process. And remember to keep windows and doors open when you cleanse, so these energies have a way to leave the space. If you are doing a ritual around letting go, then make sure you cleanse at the end too, or you can have a bowl of Palo Santo wood burning throughout.

Connect to a Higher Power

♥

You don't have to be religious or spiritual to know that there are forces greater than ourselves that operate in our lives. When we do these rituals, we want to connect to whatever the higher power is that we feel most comfortable with. It might be Nature, Life-force, the Heart, Ancestors, a Greater Intelligence, the Universe, God. You can call upon this higher power in your rituals simply by asking for their support and feeling their guidance in your body.

Dedicate to the Highest Good

♥

Whatever we are hoping to manifest through these rituals, whether it's letting go of some old pain or bringing in more love and abundance, we should always dedicate the ritual to the Highest Good. This core intention helps to ensure that the magic of ritual is used in a harmonious way, for the benefit of all beings everywhere.

Gratitude

♥

Always come back to a space of gratitude at the end of the ritual. Gratitude is the Master Key that unlocks so many wonderful things in our lives, so it's a good idea to close each ritual by expressing thanks.

Morning Rituals

'I have always been delighted at the
prospect of a new day, a fresh try ...
with perhaps a bit of magic waiting
somewhere behind the morning.'

J. B. Priestley, *Delight*

4

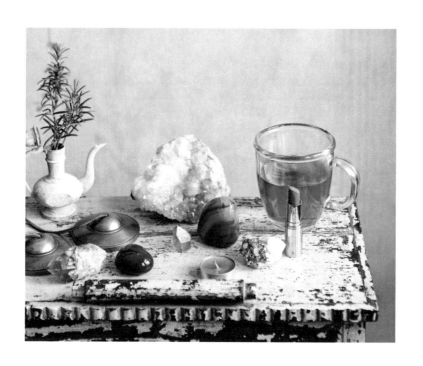

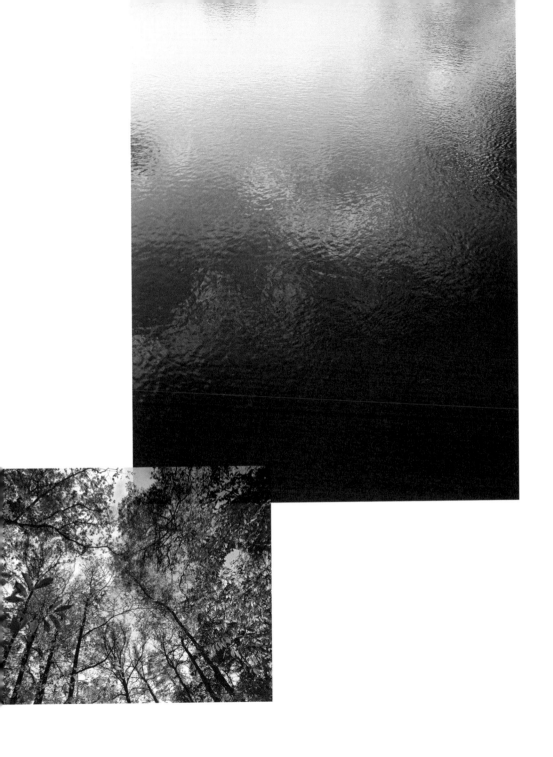

Waking Up

If we wake up in the right way, we can sprinkle magic into our day. But of course, some mornings can feel like a struggle. Maybe you aren't a great sleeper, maybe you hit the snooze button a few times, desperately squeezing a few extra minutes in bed, or maybe you have kids, pets or loud neighbours and you start the day grumpy, your beauty sleep disrupted by something out of your control. Anthony De Mello tells a wonderful story from a Spanish TV show about a man knocking on his son's door:

'Jaime,' he says. 'Wake up!'

Jaime answers, 'I don't want to get up, Papa.'

The father shouts, 'Get up, you have to go to school.'

Jaime says, 'But I don't want to go to school today.'

'Why not?' asks the father.

'Three reasons,' says Jaime. 'First, because it's so boring; second, the kids are not very nice to me; and third, I hate school.'

And the father says, 'Well, I'm going to give you three reasons why you must go to school. First, because it is your duty; second, because you're forty-five years old; and third, because you are the headmaster.'

Whether you're a 'morning person' or not, you might already have your own routines that help to get you ready for the day ahead. Some people get up and go to the gym, some do yoga, others like a nice cup of coffee. Most women will have a beauty routine, putting their 'face' on for the day ahead; many of us will reach over and turn on our phones or computers, instantly opening our minds to a whole world of information, news and work-stresses. But often these routines can feel robotic, like we're on autopilot. If our mornings start out on autopilot, it's very likely our days will continue in a mindless and reactive way. And, as Annie Dillard says, 'How we spend our days is, of course, how we spend our lives.'

Mindful morning rituals are a way to infuse beauty, intention and magic into your morning routine, and indeed into your whole life.

One of the key questions that you'll need to keep asking yourself as you move deeper into morning rituals is simply this:

HOW DO I WANT TO BE TODAY?

Introduction to Morning Rituals

The following are some general tips that will help you to wake up in the right way. Don't worry, you don't need to do it all at once. You can just choose one of these practices to start with, and build from there.

FIRST MOMENTS OF WAKING UP

Whilst we sleep and our bodies are all snuggled up in bed, our minds can travel to other worlds, where they dance with different emotions and experiences. If we wake up and reach straight for our devices without giving space to process these energies, we can find ourselves distracted and burdened throughout the day. Tristan Harris, former ethical designer at Google, explains that the act of looking at our phone first thing in the morning 'frames the experience of "waking up in the morning" around a menu of "all the things I've missed since yesterday".' This can create anxiety, and we don't want to start our day in an anxious state of being.

So, adding mindfulness and a splash of Inner Beauty to the first moments of waking up sets us up properly for the day ahead.

It helps to become mindful of the first thoughts that surface in the morning, as these can have a big influence on our day. One way I like to become mindful of my first thoughts is by changing my body posture, sitting upright or on the edge of my bed, and just taking a brief moment to check in with my mind. Sometimes, I'll hold a crystal taken from my bedside table. I also love waking up with a splash of Agua de Florida in my hands to cultivate mindfulness; the lavender and clove notes instantly bring me into presence. If there are any disharmonious thoughts first thing in the morning, I notice them with loving awareness, let them go, and then bring to mind a couple of things I'm grateful for from the last twenty-four hours. Next time you wake up, see what a difference it makes to your day if you take just a moment to focus on what you want to give thanks for. If you have a partner, it can be nice to wake up with this gratitude practice done together.

The first practical step I take once I get out of bed is to open the bedroom window, letting in the fresh air and welcoming in the new day. This might be something you already do anyway, but you can enhance this action by doing it with an extra bit of mindfulness: by opening the window we give the old, stale, unwanted energies from the night a way out and we welcome in the fresh air and the energy of the morning sun. In many Native and South American traditions, facing directly to the sun in the morning is the ultimate act of respect for this life-sustaining star. If you've ever done yoga, you'll know a similar Vedic tradition of greeting the sun in the morning: the set of poses known as the 'sun-salutation'.

With the window open, the bedroom is now ready for us to cleanse any heavy energy, especially if we've had a bad dream. I like to keep a bit of Palo Santo wood or sage in my bedroom. As I burn the smudging tool, I walk around the bedroom and visualize the energy floating out of the room along with the smoke. I also thank the spirit of the smudging plant I'm working with. You can use whatever affirmations, blessings or prayers you feel moved to in this morning cleansing ritual. The most important thing is that you allow the words to arise spontaneously from your heart, so that your smudging doesn't turn into just another robotic routine.

NURTURING YOUR SACRED SPACE IN THE MORNING

**'Arranging a bowl of flowers in the morning can give a sense of
quiet in a crowded day – like writing a poem or saying a prayer.'**
Anne Morrow Lindbergh, *Gift From the Sea*

Spending time nurturing and connecting with my sacred space is a big part of
my morning Inner Beauty practice. Remember, your sacred space is a garden for
growing your inner goddess. To wake up my inner goddess, I like to make sure the
flowers in my sacred space are fresh and the plants are watered. I burn some sage
or Palo Santo wood to clean the energy, and change some of the crystals if I'm
feeling more of a connection to a different kind of quality. You might like to check
in with the objects in your sacred space to see which ones feel right, which ones
are bringing you joy this morning. Pull those that bring you joy more into view. If
you feel you want to connect with a certain vibe it can help to write the relevant
word or phrase on a piece of paper and set this in your sacred space as a reminder.

WATER BLESSING

Water is often the first thing we reach for when we wake up. But water in the
morning is so much more than a rehydration tool; it is a sacred element, honoured
and celebrated in many different traditions. It is the blood that runs through the
veins of Mother Earth. Water is the sustainer of life. The human body consists
of 85 per cent water. It is so essential, but it's also so easily taken for granted,
especially if we have clean running water. When I recently visited Isla del Sol
in Bolivia, the water supply was carried up the mountain to our guest-house by
donkeys! Every drop was precious. Taking a little time each day to honour water
is a perfect way to bring mindfulness, beauty and gratitude into your morning
routine. So how do we honour water? Well, I learned from my Native and South
American teachers that we can speak our prayers and intentions directly into
water. Just before I gulp down my morning dose, I try to remember to speak my
gratitude or intention into the water. As I drink, I feel the water flowing around
my body with the energy of this intention. To add an extra element of kind-
hearted reciprocity (*ayni*), you can pour the last bit of water into the earth (onto
a plant or flower, or into the ground if you have a garden).

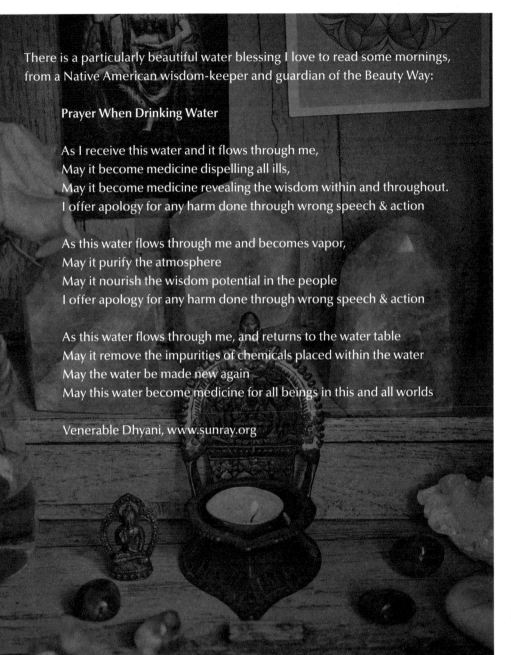

There is a particularly beautiful water blessing I love to read some mornings, from a Native American wisdom-keeper and guardian of the Beauty Way:

Prayer When Drinking Water

As I receive this water and it flows through me,
May it become medicine dispelling all ills,
May it become medicine revealing the wisdom within and throughout.
I offer apology for any harm done through wrong speech & action

As this water flows through me and becomes vapor,
May it purify the atmosphere
May it nourish the wisdom potential in the people
I offer apology for any harm done through wrong speech & action

As this water flows through me, and returns to the water table
May it remove the impurities of chemicals placed within the water
May the water be made new again
May this water become medicine for all beings in this and all worlds

Venerable Dhyani, www.sunray.org

YOUR SACRED MORNING BEAUTY ROUTINE

For many of us an important part of our morning routine is applying make-up, which helps us feel more confident and ready for the day. On some mornings time is of the essence, and I'm often amazed to see women on their way to work on the busy Underground skilfully applying full make-up in challenging circumstances. But for mornings when we do have more time, there is something magical about sprinkling a little Inner Beauty ritual into your normal routine. It's like glitter for your Third Eye!

First I like to make sure my dressing table (or wherever I'm doing my make-up) is an inviting and sacred space by placing it next to natural light, adding crystals, plants, flowers and an oilburner or scented candle. Placed in view, I have an image of a goddess to remind me of the Divine Feminine qualities I want to tap into (I personally love Tara, the Buddhist goddess, as she is a symbol of peace and unity. But you can choose whichever feminine form inspires you the most: it could be a female artist, a spiritual teacher, or your mother or grandmother).

Sometimes, it's not easy to tap into the Divine Feminine during our morning beauty routine. I know for myself that when my skin's been playing up, or I've not had enough sleep and I've got dark circles under my eyes, I look at my reflection in the mirror and can be harshly critical of my appearance, zooming in on the bits I don't like! Whenever I catch myself in this self-critical headspace, I take an 'Inner Beauty Pause', because I know this negative mind-chatter can easily dominate my thoughts and feelings throughout the day if I don't address it. Remember, beauty is so much more than skin-deep, and these moments when we catch ourselves lost in self-judgement really do contain huge potential for the cultivation of Inner Beauty. Within the Inner Beauty Pause, I take a deep breath in and visualize breathing out any heavy, critical energy. I then bring my attention to something about myself I know I can feel positive about (it doesn't need to be physical, it can be a personal quality or an act of kindness you've done recently or plan to do that day). Once I've refocussed my attention towards appreciation, I then allow myself to embrace my imperfections, in the spirit of *wabi-sabi*. (See the Ageing Ritual on page 187 for more inspiration.) As you practise the Inner Beauty Pause, you are training your mind and heart to embrace your whole self, including your 'imperfections'. If you're up for a really strong reminder, you can write on your mirror a word or message to help remember your Inner Beauty: one such beautiful message is simply 'I am enough'.

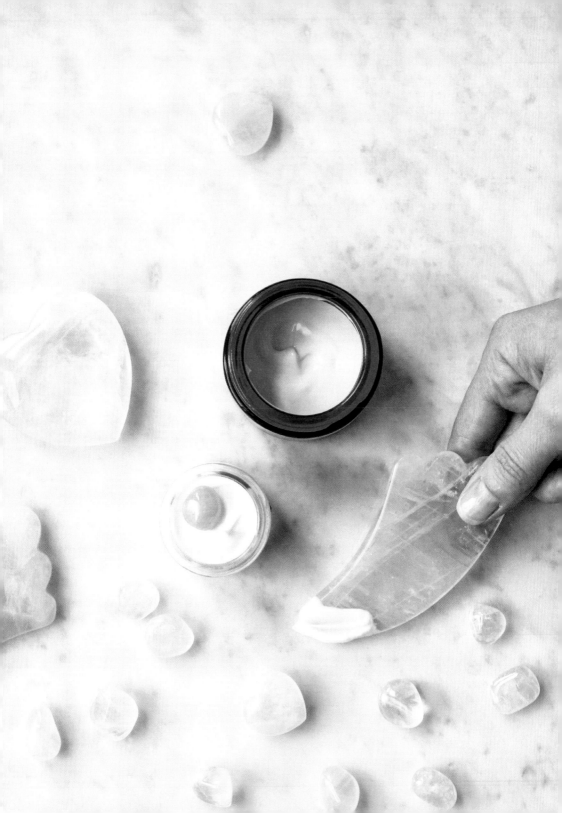

Earlier in the crystal section, I shared that the living goddesses of Ancient Egypt would add powdered Rose Quartz into their beauty potions to prevent wrinkles and restore a glowing complexion. So, how can we modern girls tap into these ancient beauty practices of our sister goddesses? Well, one way I particularly love is using a Rose Quartz tool to apply my face cream. Using this tool to massage cream into the skin will help blood flow circulation, bringing a glow back to the skin. The tool I use is a palm-size, smooth and flattish stone, so application is easy. You might want to take some time to search for a particular shape, size or smoothness of stone that feels right for you.

Cleansing the energy of your tool beforehand (using your favourite cleansing tool), and with gratitude and respect, take your Rose Quartz beauty tool, dip it into the cream, then use it to mindfully massage the cream into your face. Whilst doing this, I visualize my face glowing with a delicate pink light, restoring my inner and outer beauty. When the weather is hot, I keep my Rose Quartz tool in the fridge overnight so that in the morning it refreshes my skin and helps tighten my pores.

For on-the-go beauty, I love to add one or two small crystal tumble stones into the cream itself – whether face or body cream. Before dunking them in, make sure you've cleansed and blessed the stones. The wonderful thing about doing this is that it naturally infuses your everyday creams with crystal magic, and also allows you to personalize your sacred beauty ritual to your skin's needs. For example, if I'm feeling my skin needs an energizing boost, I'll add some Carnelian or clear Quartz, to help relax I'll add Amethyst, and to nurture I'll add Rose Quartz.

'But for mornings when we do have more time, there is something magical about sprinkling a little Inner Beauty ritual into your normal routine. It's like glitter for your Third Eye!'

The Morning Rituals

In this section, you'll find some specific morning rituals that can help you tune into and manifest particular Inner Beauty energies or qualities in your day. I really encourage you to get creative and play around with the ideas here to see what works best for you.

Remember, the key question running through all of these rituals is simply: 'How do I want to be today?'

The clearer a picture you can have in your heart of how you want to be, the more powerful the ritual will be for you.

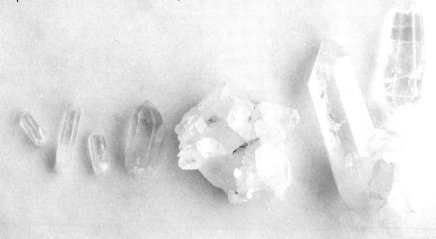

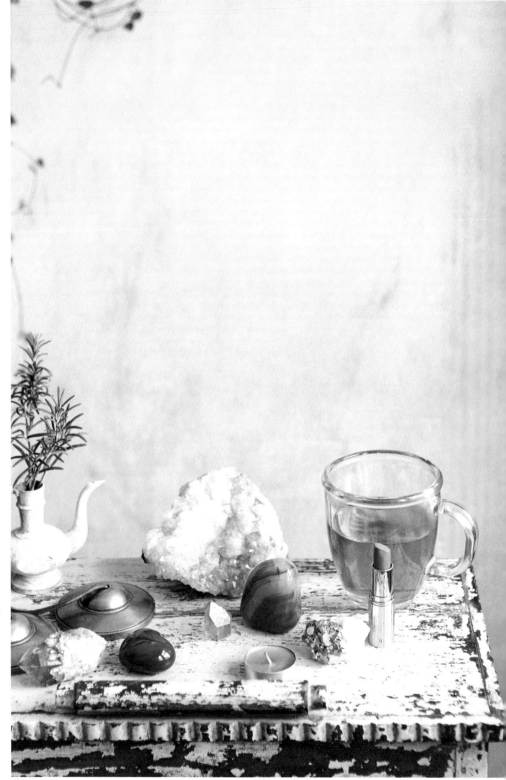
Morning Rituals

'You have a phenomenal amount of energy inside you.
The only reason you don't feel this energy ... is because you block it.'
Michael Singer

Energy is infinite, if you know how to channel it. Just take a moment to think back to the last time you had some good news out of the blue. Notice how you suddenly got an energy-boost, how your whole being felt alive and vibrant. The really, really good news is that you can channel this infinite supply of energy without needing to wait for some positive event to happen in the outside world. The following ritual will help you to achieve this. This ritual is particularly good for when you're feeling tired, unmotivated, and you really want or need a boost of energy, putting a spring in your step.

Ingredients

- Plant or flowers
- Agua de Florida or energizing essential oil such as orange, black pepper, basil or ginger
- Yellow or gold candle
- Carnelian or clear Quartz stone
- Bright lipstick or nail polish

Prepare the space to welcome energy in

The first step is to make sure that the space you're going to do the ritual in is organized, free of any clutter, and makes you feel energized. We all know how energized we can feel after a good spring clean. Energy flows around a room, especially from windows and doors, so it can really help to move any obstacles blocking this flow. We also want to have flourishing plants or flowers to represent the energy of life. You will need some Agua de Florida (or some other energizing fragrance), a candle (preferably yellow or gold) and a Carnelian or clear Quartz stone. Once you have the space ready, give the space, your tools and yourself a good energetic cleanse with your favourite smudging tool.

Connect to presence through smell

Once your space is ready for an energy-boost, splash some Agua de Florida into your cupped hands, rub your hands together, hold them over your nose and breathe in the revitalizing fragrance, then move your hands around your body, imagining every cell in your body coming fully alive in a beautiful harmonious inner smile.

Light a candle

I like to light a yellow or gold candle as this colour connects me to the infinite energy of the sun. You can choose a candle in a colour that represents energy-boosting for you.

Set your intention

Now you are ready to get a very clear answer to the following question:

'What will I do with this extra energy I'm cultivating today?'

Take a minute to close your eyes and visualize each step of your day ahead. Get a clear picture of how you will serve yourself and the world with all this extra energy you're about to channel. What will you create? What positive effect will this extra energy have on yourself? And what positive effect will this energy have on other people you come into contact with today?

Energizing blessing

Now take the Carnelian or clear Quartz stone in your hand. With the stone in my hand, I like to say the following blessing (but you can say whatever feels right in your heart): 'I open up and welcome the infinite supply of energy that is available to me throughout this day, always for the highest good.'

Candle-flame energy visualization

Now for my favourite part of this ritual. Cast your gaze at the candle flame, and then close your eyes and imagine that flame is flickering inside your being. With each flicker, feel the flame burning away any heavy energy, worries, tiredness, tension or limiting beliefs, allowing pure, refined energy (*sami*) to circulate freely around your body and mind. As you do this, feel your back straighten as you start to feel stronger. You can return to this inner image of the candle flame and the sense of abundant energy at any time during the day.

Close the ritual

To bring this ritual to an end, I blow the candle out and then I take a moment to give thanks for this precious reminder that energy is infinite, and the flame within burns bright and eternal.

♥ Extra touches

There are a couple of extra touches I sometimes add here. For one, I like to place the Carnelian or clear Quartz stone into a glass of water or portable water filter. The stone will infuse the water with its energy. I also like to keep a Carnelian stone on me, so I can place it in the space where I'm working that day. Another really nice touch to give you a boost is to wear a bright lipstick or nail polish or more brightly coloured clothes. The great thing about this is that the bright colours will act as a reminder of your energy intention every time you look down at your hands or look in the mirror.

**'Concentrate all your thoughts upon the work at hand.
The sun's rays do not burn until brought to a focus.'**
Alexander Graham Bell

In today's age of distraction, focus can be hard to achieve. The internet, our digital devices, our emails and social media accounts, are all constantly chipping away at our ability to focus. The average attention span in 2013 was down – from twelve seconds in 2000 – to eight seconds, less than that of a goldfish at nine seconds. Are you still with me? Don't worry, you are definitely not on your own. There are some days I keep catching myself mindlessly scrolling through social media, and it can feel like such a massive effort to keep my mind on the task. And I have a feeling that focussing is only going to become more difficult as our devices get smarter, and the number of apps we use continues to multiply. And yet, focus is one of the most important skills we have. Focus allows us to zoom in on what is most important to us, so that we can create beauty in ourselves and in the world.

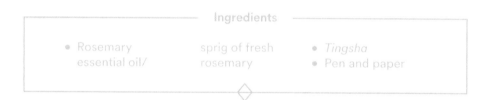

Ingredients

- Rosemary essential oil/
- sprig of fresh rosemary
- *Tingsha*
- Pen and paper

Prepare the space for focus
Start this ritual by taking some time to mindfully tidy up any clutter around your ritual space. A clean and tidy space supports a clean and tidy mind.

Declutter your mind
Take a piece of paper and a pen and simply write down as many things as you can that have been distracting you recently. It might be certain thoughts, it might be conversations, it might be all the outstanding tasks on your to-do list. Don't think too hard: just put pen to paper and start writing freely, letting the words naturally flow out from your mind on to the piece of paper. Keep going

until you feel lighter and have a good sense that you have decluttered your mind. When you reach this point and are starting to feel more clear and focussed, rip that piece of paper up into as many pieces as you can. At this point, I like to sound my *tingsha*, moving the instrument over the top of the ripped pieces of paper, to cleanse away these distractions and to welcome the energy of focus into the ritual space. Place the ripped paper now to one side out of view, remembering to dispose of the pieces after the ritual is over.

Cultivate focus with rosemary oil and Clear Quartz

Now you have decluttered your mind, add a couple of drops of rosemary oil to your fingertips and massage the essence into your earlobes. This is a wonderful technique from the Ayurvedic sciences. The ears are connected to the brain, and specifically to mental clarity, whilst rosemary is itself really effective for bringing clarity of mind and focus. With each mindful movement around your earlobe, feel your mind getting sharper and more focussed. If you'd like to add an extra touch here, you can move this fragrance around your body with your hands, creating a kind of force field of focus.

Now take a Clear Quartz stone and a sprig of rosemary into your hand. Clear Quartz is known to help amplify energy and cultivate focus. Close your eyes and bring to mind one important goal that you want to achieve today. Make sure the goal is realistic, achievable and fulfilling. Bring to mind the reason why this goal is so important to you (a clear motivation is very important to aid focus). Finally, visualize yourself at the end of the day feeling really happy that you have achieved your goal with perfect focus and clarity.

Now blow a sacred breath into the stone, thanking the stone for supporting you with all the focus you need to achieve this goal today. (This sacred breath practice is inspired by Andean tradition, where intentions are blown into the sacred coca leaf as part of a *despacho*.)

End and bring focus with you

Your Quartz is now ready to be your focus buddy today. I recommend carrying the Clear Quartz around with you throughout the day, placing it in view on your workspace. Before finishing, I like to sound the *tingsha* again to cleanse the space and bring this ritual to an end. Sometimes, I'll bring the sprig of rosemary with me and keep it with my Clear Quartz on my desk.

♥

'Your heart knows the way. Run in that direction.'
Rumi

Of all the places I connect with in my morning rituals, the heart is right at the top of my list. Heart is the sacred well from which the highest Inner Beauty qualities are drawn. When I'm connected with my heart, I'm naturally more compassionate, more grateful, more kind, more appreciative of the beauty within and around me. It's no surprise that the heart lies at the centre of so many different spiritual traditions. The spiritual heart is the antidote to our busy, anxious, judging minds. A great Indian saint, Nisargadatta, sums this up beautifully: 'The mind creates the abyss, the heart crosses it.' Where the mind worries, the heart trusts. Where the mind is divisive, the heart unifies. When your heart is singing in love with the world, then the mind has no choice but to be quiet.

It's definitely not always easy to stay connected to the heart. Our hearts get hurt from time to time. And when our hearts get hurt, we tend to contract, crawling back into our protective shells. Every single day, life is testing our heart's ability to stay open. Have a think now about the small, everyday things that might cause your heart to contract. Do you ever worry about what someone might be thinking about you? Do you hide from others (or even from yourself) the parts of you that you feel are not good enough? Maybe you judge yourself harshly when you act in a way that is less than beautiful, less than perfect? Are you someone who feels awkward when they receive a compliment? Being able to receive love is a big part of having an open heart.

The other side is of course being able to give love. And again, when the heart is contracted, when it feels hurt, we sometimes struggle to let love flow out into the world. Some of the most inspiring, beautiful souls I've ever met seem to have this ability to give and receive love effortlessly, like water flowing freely. And I'm sure a big reason why love flows in these people's lives is simply because they've learned to accept and love themselves first and foremost, warts and all. American therapist and spiritual teacher John Welwood talks about this need to accept all of our parts, the beauty and the beast, because then 'this beauty you are can begin to care for the beast you sometimes seem to be . . . the beast is nothing other than your wounded beauty.' In this heart ritual, my hope is that you can come to love all sides of your Nature, the dark and the light, so that your heart can remember its true purpose: 'to be an open channel through which great love flows into this world.'

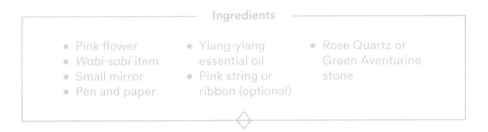

Ingredients

- Pink flower
- *Wabi-sabi* item
- Small mirror
- Pen and paper
- Ylang-ylang essential oil
- Pink string or ribbon (optional)
- Rose Quartz or Green Aventurine stone

Prepare the space for heart-opening

Beauty itself has the power to open our hearts. So, with this ritual, I really recommend taking a few mindful moments to make your ritual space beautiful. I like to scatter pink flower petals around it for that extra touch. I will also include one thing that represents *wabi-sabi*: the beauty of imperfection. It can be a chipped shell, a piece of driftwood, a decaying leaf, or any imperfect or tarnished object that your heart can connect to. I also place a hand mirror in the space. In Sufi wisdom, the heart is a polished mirror: 'You must wipe it clean of the veil of dust that has gathered upon it, because it is destined to reflect the light of divine secrets' (Sufi proverb). Once the space is prepared, as always we need to cleanse all the Inner Beauty tools, the space and ourselves.

Soften the hardness around our hearts

Before we can enter our true heart space, we need to acknowledge and soften the things that are hardening around our hearts. Bring to mind one time during the past week when you know your heart has closed up. Maybe you lost your temper, got impatient, judged someone else, struggled to forgive, experienced fear in a corner of your life, or were harsh on yourself. As you run through this moment gently in your mind, cast your gaze towards your *wabi-sabi* object, and as you appreciate its imperfect beauty, allow yourself for a moment to feel compassion for this same imperfect beauty of your own being. Then take a really deep breath in, and as you breathe out make a loud sighing noise to signify release, whilst giving your hands a really good shake, offering yourself total permission to let go of any hardness around your heart. (Letting go here does not mean we're letting go of responsibility for our actions; this action simply acknowledges that we can best learn from these moments when we don't let them harden around our hearts.)

Connect with your heart

Now take a couple of drops of ylang-ylang oil (ylang-ylang is a relaxing oil associated with the heart), gently massage it into the palm of your right hand and place your hand over the centre of your chest, your heart centre. Next, take either a Rose Quartz or a Green Aventurine stone (Green Aventurine brings balance to the heart), and hold the stone in your left hand (the side of your heart). I like to set an intention into the stone with an affirmation: 'May this stone help me polish the mirror of my heart, so that my Inner Beauty qualities can shine forth in service of Love.'

Choose your heart quality for the day

Now we have a strong connection to our heart space, it's time to decide what heart quality we want to manifest today. There are a number of different qualities associated with the heart; some of the main ones are compassion, forgiveness, gratitude, kindness and vulnerability. For each of these, you can add a 'self-', as in 'self-compassion'. Now write your chosen heart quality down, either on a small piece of paper or on the mirror, using eye liner or a dry erase pen. A lovely alternative here is to take some pink string or ribbon and tie it around your wrist as a beautiful reminder of your chosen heart quality throughout the day.

Expand light through the body

Now you have a particular heart quality in mind, with the stone still in your left hand, close your eyes and with your right hand placed over your heart centre, imagine that this sacred touch is bringing to life your chosen heart quality, beginning with a small pinprick of soft pink light at the centre of your chest. Now you can watch as this light slowly expands outwards from the centre of your chest, gently filling every cell of your being with this heart quality. When your whole body is bathed in this beautiful light, take a moment to visualize how your day will unfold as this heart quality shines brightly and effortlessly from the core of your being. Think especially of any potential challenges in your day ahead and visualize how your chosen heart quality will shine forth in these moments.

Gratitude

Now bring to mind one thing from the last twenty-four hours you can feel grateful for. Gratitude is a master at opening our hearts. It can be something small, like a nice cup of tea, or maybe someone made a small, kind gesture for you. Bring this moment to mind as though it's happening right now. Connect with the feelings of joy and appreciation in your heart. You may find that your mind naturally moves to different moments you feel grateful for. If so, it's absolutely fine: the more the merrier!

Kindness

When you've brought this moment of gratitude from the last twenty-four hours fully into your heart, bring to mind someone in your life who has been suffering recently. Sometimes, when our hearts close, we can also close ourselves off to those people we know who may need our help. Make a small commitment to do something kind for that person in the next twenty-four hours. Again, it can be something small like sending them a simple message just letting them know you're thinking about them.

simple acts of kindness

Send a message to them to thank them for being who they are, just the way they are.

Carve out some sacred time to spend with them, no distractions. Presence is the greatest gift.

Send flowers or a plant out of the blue.

Write them a heartfelt letter.

Figure out one task they really hate doing and offer to do it for them.

Close

To close this ritual, I love to spritz my face with rosewater: the sweet smell of rose brings me back into presence (and my skin gets a nice hydration boost as a little beauty bonus). I will then carry my Rose Quartz or Aventurine with me throughout the day, or, if I use the pink string or ribbon, I'll wear it on my wrist, as a reminder to stay connected to my heart-space.

♥ Extra touch

As an extra Inner Beauty heart-boost, I love to have a poem to read at the start or end of this ritual, as poetry is a direct bridge to the heart. One of my favourites for this purpose is Derek Walcott's poem, 'Love after Love'.

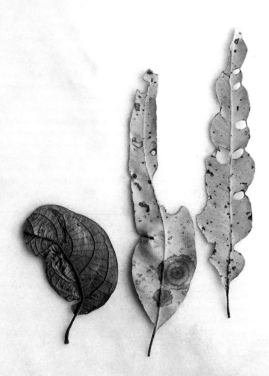

✦

'We do not attract what we want; we attract what we are.'
Wayne Dyer

This abundance ritual is perfect for mornings when you're feeling a sense of lack in some corner of your life: maybe you didn't get enough sleep, then you look in your wardrobe and can't find anything you want to wear; maybe a huge bill just arrived and your bank balance is looking a bit sad. Starting the day with a sense of lack, we can easily get trapped in a negative loop: worrying, agitated, feeling how unlucky we are, thinking life is unfair. And in the age of social media, it's all too easy to feel the grass is always greener on the other side, as you look green-eyed at pictures of beautiful beaches, fun parties, perfect homes, perfect lives.

The irony is that when we're in this scarcity state of mind we're less likely to see and embrace opportunities when they come. There's a part of our brain called the Reticular Activating System that acts like a filter. It makes sure our brain doesn't get overloaded with more information than it can handle, actively blocking from our awareness information that doesn't fit in with our current way of thinking. Think of it in the way Facebook only shows you things you've already expressed a preference for. It means that, if we start the day with a scarcity mindset, our brain-filters will only let information in that fits in with our fear-based thought process.

This is why the abundance ritual is so helpful. When we focus less on what we can get and more on what we already have to give, the universe will naturally reflect this back to us. This is a perfect example of the spirit of *ayni* (reciprocity) that the wisdom-keepers of the Andes hold in such high esteem. Even though they have fewer material possessions than people in many parts of the world, they constantly give gifts to Mother Earth in appreciation for her abundance. When we give of ourselves, this spirit is reflected by the universe as our hearts grow abundant with a deeper sense of peace and love. When we start the day with an abundance mindset it not only allows us to feel content with who we are and what we have to give, but also increases the chance that we'll attract more good stuff into our hearts and lives.

Before you start, think about your own relationship to abundance. Were you encouraged as a child to believe that life would provide what you need? How do you react to those who seem to have more than you: more status, more money, more happiness?

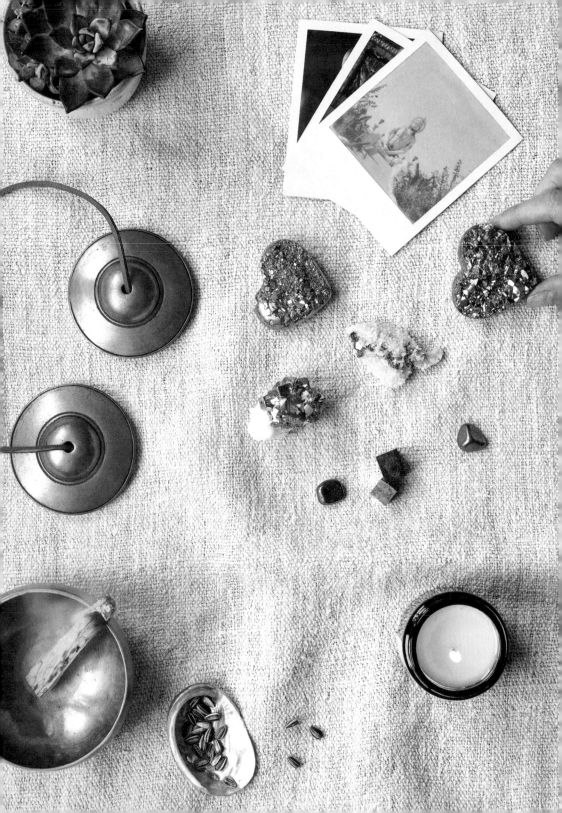

- Pen and paper
- Citrine stone
- Plant
- Musical instrument

Suggestions for
Abundance Corner:
- Seeds
- Luxury candle

- Photos of happy
  memories/places
  you want to visit
- Pyrite crystal

Prepare a space for abundance

If possible, I really recommend having a separate corner in your home that is dedicated to abundance. If this isn't possible, then simply dedicate one part of your sacred space or even a little space on a shelf to manifesting abundance. In this corner, we want to inspire feelings of plenty, of luxury, of inspiration, of life and growth. I like to keep lush plants, flowers, seeds, pictures of places I want to visit, a photo of a happy memory, a luxury candle, a small musical instrument to welcome in joy. I also keep a Pyrite crystal in this space (Pyrite looks like gold, with the same sense of luxurious beauty, and is known to support abundance). Have a think about what objects would symbolize abundance for you. Add these objects to your abundance corner where possible. When your corner is ready, you can give yourself, the space and the tools a good energetic cleanse.

Remove blockages to abundance

Now we have a space prepared for abundance, we need to acknowledge any places where we're feeling a lack in our lives. We're going to see if there are any fears that might be holding us back. I remember a period in my make-up career when the work quite suddenly dried up and I definitely had some worries, questioning my value and my skills, wondering if I could even make it into a career at all. It was an unsettling time, but then I remember moving into a new flat and creating a sacred space with a beautiful abundance corner. At the same time, my husband helped me to see that I was holding on to some limiting beliefs (these are the moments when it's quite handy to have a partner who's a therapist!). I managed to turn these limiting thoughts into an abundance mindset. It wasn't long before I found one of the best clients I've ever worked with, and shortly afterwards I set up The Colourful Dot, which was a dream creative project that opened up so many other opportunities, including writing this book right now!

The first step is to choose one area where you feel a lack (e.g. money, health, relationships, happiness, time, fulfilment) and write this one word down at the top of a piece of paper.

Now sit by your abundance corner or in any quiet space

Close your eyes and bring to mind the one word that you wrote at the top of your piece of paper. Notice what thoughts and feelings come up for you when you hold this word in mind. Pay close attention to any fearful thoughts, nervous energy or a sinking feeling in your heart. Explore if there are any patterns that recur in your life where you might be missing opportunities to give or receive because of your scarcity mindset in this area.

It's time to remove these fear-based blockages to abundance

Light a smudging tool and move it mindfully around your whole body, giving yourself total permission to let go of any blockages to abundance.

Unlock the abundance mindset

Now comes the fun part! Take your piece of paper and complete the following affirmations as they relate to your chosen subject: *one way in which I would act differently in my life if I knew deep down that I had as much X as I need is …* If you want to take this deeper, beneath this write down: *one way in which I would share my gift with the world more effectively if I knew that I had as much X as I need is …*

Visualize abundance

When you've written these abundance statements down, take a piece of Citrine (stone of abundance) in your hand, close your eyes again, and spend some time gently visualizing the things you'll do with the abundance available to you. Connect in your heart with the feelings of joy associated with this abundance. Whilst tracing the outline of your abundance, leave some space for the unexpected, as this keeps you open to magical synchronicities in your life. Make one commitment to something you will do in the next twenty-four hours as a result of your abundance in this chosen area of your life (perhaps it's something you have been putting off because of your scarcity mindset). This part of the ritual is so important. We often put so many things off because of our scarcity mindset, because we fear we don't have enough of something to be ready. British actor/comedian Hugh Laurie says: 'It's a terrible thing, I think, in life to wait until you're ready. I have this feeling now that actually no one is ever ready to do anything. There is almost no such thing as ready. There is only now. And you may as well do it now. Generally speaking, now is as good a time as any.'

Grow abundance
When you're ready, place the piece of paper in the soil of a plant, and place this plant in your abundance area. This is so that your dreams can manifest as the plant grows. I also like to keep my Citrine with me during the day as a reminder of the abundance I am manifesting.

Nurture an abundance mindset
Our intentions naturally change, so it's important to revisit this ritual and the abundance statements on the piece of paper you've planted. You can keep refining, updating and changing these statements. The important thing is that you're revisiting and strengthening the feeling of abundance each time you reconnect. Whenever you water the plant, give gratitude for the abundance the universe or Mother Earth is providing for you, and for the highest good of all beings.

Evening/
Night-time
Rituals

'No more words.
In the name of this place we
drink in with our breathing,
stay quiet like a flower.
So the nightbirds
will start singing.'

Rumi

5

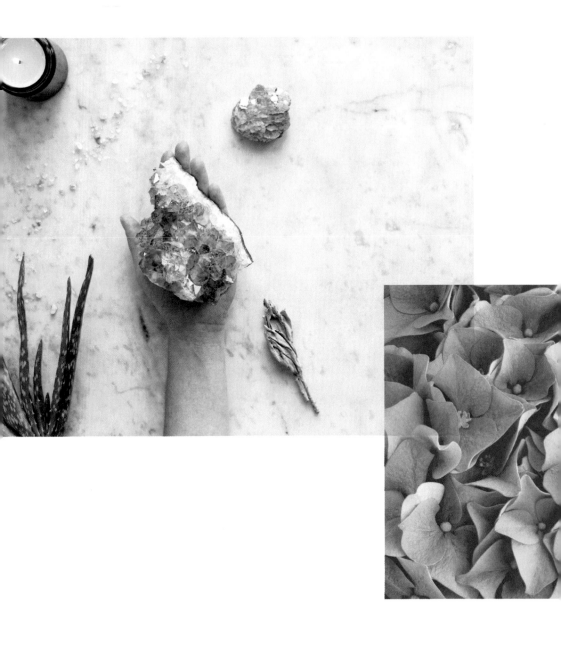

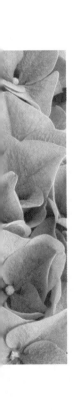

Winding Down

Traditionally, the evening was a time to wind down from the day's work, eat good food, hang out with family and friends, and get your body ready for a peaceful night of beauty sleep. In the olden days with no electric lighting, a natural process of unwinding occurred as the sun would set and the body relaxed. These days, the distinction between day and night and between work and rest has definitely become more blurred. I often work from home, so I really do know how difficult it can be to officially stop the working day and start the evening's relaxation. The temptation to check my work emails is always lurking. And this temptation carries on well into the evening and bedtime when I should really be unwinding in preparation for my beauty sleep. Even when we're doing something relaxing (having a bath, watching TV, eating a nice dinner), the temptation to be online, to be connected, and to respond is ever present. It's as though the addictive allure of our online worlds and the fear of missing out now have more power over our choices than the desire to look after ourselves and to properly relax.

How relaxed do you normally feel when you climb into bed? When was the last time you had a really good night's sleep? And how did you feel in the morning?

A super-simple tip to get you started with evening rituals is to use a smudging tool when you've decided to bring your working day to an end. As soon as I finish my working day, I reach for my Palo Santo stick and cleanse away any lingering energies, feeling a sense of freshness and renewal as I breathe in the scent, and consciously welcome in a phase of rest and relaxation.

I have a 'prayer plant' at home in my bedroom (*Maranta leuconeura*), which is my personal daily reminder of how to balance work and rest. When the sun sets, the leaves of the plant mark the end of their day by folding together, like hands closed in prayer. Then, in the morning, the leaves unfurl towards the light of the morning sun. When I see the leaves closed in prayer in the evenings, it instantly softens my mind and body as though my natural need to unwind is activated. I hope that in a similar way doing these rituals can help you to make your evenings/night-times into a time of sanctuary, a time to really nourish and restore your inner goddess, so that in the morning you are fully recharged and can rise and shine your light into the world.

'It's as though the addictive allure of our online worlds and the fear of missing out now have more power over our choices than the desire to look after ourselves and to properly relax.'

Gratitude Ritual for Your Evening Meal

'Gratitude unlocks the fullness of life … It can turn a meal into a feast, a house into a home, a stranger into a friend.'
Melody Beattie, *Codependent No More*

Evening mealtimes provide a perfect opportunity to remember the practice of gratitude. Of course, throughout history so many religions, wisdom traditions and cultures have taken a pause before eating to say thanks for the food on the plate. In parts of the Philippines, they even do a little gratitude dance, imitating a rooster scratching the ground. The purpose of these gratitude rituals is simply to help us appreciate our food by taking a little time to think about the incredible journey the food has been on before arriving on our plate. In the modern day, many of us have lost touch with this simple practice of gratitude as our food comes in packages and we usually take for granted the effort and life that brought us this gift. A major bonus of gratitude around mealtimes is that it helps to rebalance our relationship with food, especially with stress eating. Did you know that when we are stressed the taste buds that detect very sweet and very savoury foods get activated, meaning we are drawn to stuffing ourselves with chocolate and cheese? This ritual helps to retrain our brains to remember that eating is a time for de-stressing and heart-connection.

Prepare the space

Maybe you already have a fruit bowl at the centre of your dining table. It can be fun to add some extra sacred elements around this, like crystals, a plant, a candle, making a beautiful centrepiece to remind you of the sacred abundance of Mother Earth. I particularly like Rose Quartz (for loving connections), Blue Lace Agate (for calm energy and good communication), and some Pyrite or Citrine (for abundance), but you can use whatever crystals feel right for you. You might want to have a specific gratitude blessing framed on the wall in this area too.

Gratitude Food Blessing

In this ritual, before anyone starts eating we give thanks for the food on our plate. There are so many ways to give thanks; I encourage you to find a way that feels right for you. Even just a simple 'thank you' will help to cultivate gratitude. Eckhart Tolle says, 'If the only prayer you ever say is "Thank You", that will be enough.' When my husband and I have guests over, we like to start by holding hands to establish our connection with each other. If I'm eating alone, I like to place my right hand over my heart, close my eyes and give thanks for the food, for the journey it's been on to arrive on my plate, and for the higher power that has provided this food. This higher power can be whatever you believe in: Nature, Life, Pachamama, The Universe, God. I personally feel a strong connection to Mother Earth so I give specific thanks for her abundance. If you are eating outside, it can also be nice to show *ayni* (reciprocity) by pouring a drop of water back to Mother Earth in thanks. Or if indoors, use a houseplant.

Mindful First Mouthful

Once you've connected to that space of gratitude for the food, make the first mouthful a mindful one. When you have loaded up your first fork or spoon, slow right down, notice the colour and texture of the food, bring it to your nose and smell the food, then chew the food slowly, connecting as much as possible with the flavours in your mouth. I also like to imagine that the food I'm eating is filling my body with the energy and love of Mother Earth.

Share Appreciation

Another layer you can add to give this ritual more depth simply involves each person at the table sharing one thing they are grateful for from the day just gone. If you are eating on your own, you can just think about this one thing and take a little time to connect with the feelings of appreciation in your heart. Gratitude can make us feel 'full' in our hearts in the same way we feel full in our stomachs after a nourishing meal. This gratitude sharing can be a really fun exercise to do as a family too, especially if it's kept light-hearted and playful.

Nurturing Ritual

'Take rest; a field that has rested gives a bountiful crop.'
Ovid

Inner beauty is only possible if we make time to give back to and nurture ourselves. The evenings are the ideal time for us to replenish and restore, but this is easier said than done. We can have so many other things competing for our attention in the evenings (partners, kids, pets, work emails, house chores, to-do lists). And sometimes deep inside we may not even feel like we deserve to give back to ourselves. I find these words from poet C. Joybell C. to be so true: 'You can be the most beautiful person in the world but if you yourself don't know it, all of that doesn't even matter.' So, an essential Inner Beauty skill is the ability to create the desire, the time and the space to give back to ourselves. This ritual contains some magical ideas for that sacred 'me' time, providing a way to offer healing to yourself in the spirit of the Native American 'Beauty Way' we mentioned earlier.

Ingredients

- Mangano Calcite stone
- Rose Quartz stone
- Shells

- Pink lotus, Frankincense or rose oil
- Hand cream

- Pen and paper
- Scented candle
- Chimes

Prepare nurturing tools to support you

Mangano Calcite, with its beautiful pastel pink tones and nurturing and soothing energy, is one crystal that I love to have near me or to hold when I do this ritual, or generally whenever I'm feeling the need for soft, comforting, motherly energy. Rose Quartz, the 'Divine Mother' of crystals, is of course also a lovely stone to use here. This is a perfect time for you to select objects that represent nurture to you. I like to add some special shells. For example, I have some beautiful shells from a trip to Sri Lanka when I spent the day with a school of Buddhist Monks in a peaceful cove, mindfully picking shells on the beach. Maybe you too have some objects from a time that felt very relaxing and nurturing for you?

Prepare your nurture space

The first practical step is to create a 'do not disturb' zone for as long as you think you need. If you live with others, you might want to put a notice on the door, and simply explain to them that you need a bit of 'me' time. Next, cleanse the space with a smudging tool of your choice, and create a relaxing ambience, maybe dimming the lights, lighting a nice candle. I like to use a softly scented candle to get in the mood. You might like to surround yourself with soft, puffed-up cushions, creating a beautiful snuggle space for yourself.

Create a self-care list

The first time you do this ritual, take some time to create a self-care list. What kind of things come to mind when you really think about giving back to and nurturing yourself?

Make a list now of five ways in which you can be kinder to yourself.

My list often has a lot of pampering activities like doing a nice face-mask, painting my nails, going for a massage, eating delicious, healthy food. Once you get into the habit of focussing your mind and heart on self-care, you will find that you start to feel more gentle tenderness and compassion for yourself.

Welcome in Motherly Energy

We all have a nurturing, caring, motherly energy that we can tap into when we want some self-love. One of my favourite ways of welcoming in this energy is by using a sacred sound instrument like the Koshi chimes. The Koshi chimes are a set of other-worldly wind-chime instruments that play a sweet and soothing lullaby that is instantly relaxing. During a full moon ceremony I recently held, I loved a friend's description of the sound of these chimes as being like the sound you imagine stars would make if only you could hear them. You can use other sacred sound instruments, wind-chimes or just some nice relaxing music. I like to close my eyes and move the chimes around my body, opening myself up to receive the self-care that I need. Receiving really is a sacred act, as important as giving when done with an open heart. An extra little touch I sometimes add here is to take the Mangano Calcite in my hand, close my eyes and think about a time when I felt really nurtured and safe. It might be a time spent in Nature, on holiday, or in the presence of your family, a good friend, or a particularly loving person you know.

Pampering hand/wrist massage

Now we are open to receive, we can really get started showing ourselves some love. When I think about pampering myself, I tend to think about having a nice soak in a bath (more on this overleaf), or about having a relaxing massage. But of course, we don't always have the time or the money to go out and get a massage whenever we'd like to. Massaging our hands or wrists is a really simple and delightful way to pamper ourselves. If, like me, you're constantly putting on hand cream to combat dry hands, this hand massage is really just a more heart-centred version of that self-care routine, simply infused with a few drops of oil and an extra dash of mindful self-loving. So squeeze some hand cream into your palm and add a couple of drops of an oil that carries nurturing energy. Some of my favourite oils to use are Pink Lotus (to enhance love and serenity), Rose Absolute (for heart-connection and balance), or Frankincense (for deep relaxation). As you massage this nurture potion into your hands and wrists, be mindful of the relaxing feelings and notice the stresses dissolve away from your body and out through your fingertips.

Nurture the soul

After the massage, another step towards self-nurture is to take a few moments to read or listen to some words of wisdom from a favourite teacher, poet, singer or writer. I love to read or listen to the words of Ram Dass, Wayne Dyer, Marianne Williamson, and I really love *Oprah's Soul Series* interviews. Listening or reading to even just a few words is sometimes enough to give our soul a deep sense of nourishment.

Make a mini-commitment to self-care

To finish off this ritual, take the list you made at the start of ways you can be kinder to yourself and choose one that you can commit to doing for yourself over the next week. To help you remember these commitments, keep this list on the mirror where you do your morning beauty routine, or at the front of your diary, or on your fridge.

'Receiving really
is a sacred act, as
important as giving
when done with
an open heart.'

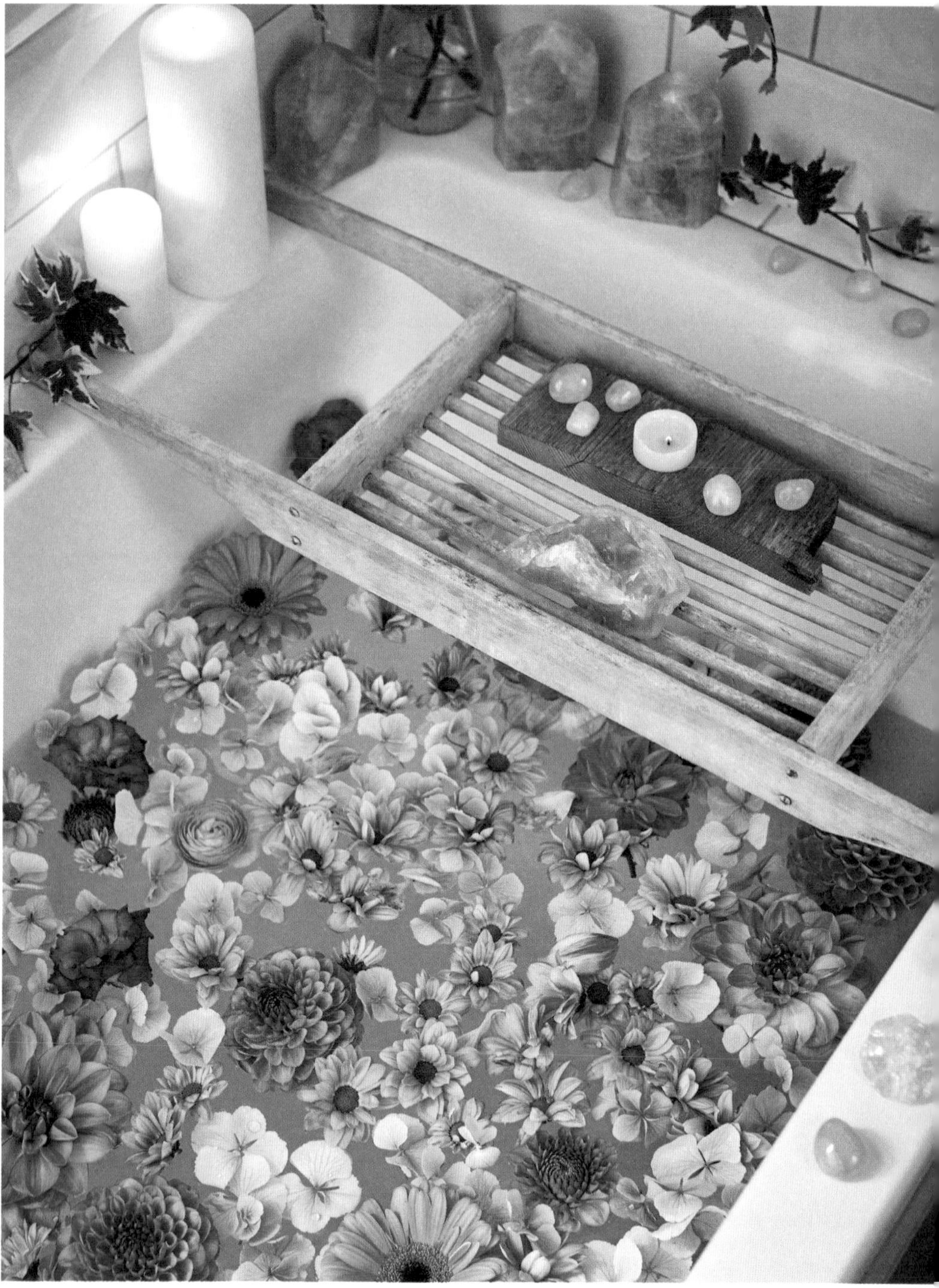

Rose Quartz Bathtime Ritual

🔹

'The supreme goodness is like water,
Which nourishes all things without trying.'
Tao Te Ching

Bathtime is sacred to me. It's often the best or only chance I have in a busy day to properly unwind. Even when I've lived in places where there was no bathtub, or the bathroom was in need of some serious TLC, I've always tried to turn this room into a sacred sanctuary, surrounding the bath with crystals, flowers, incense and candles. Many ancient cultures treated bathing as a sacred healing art. These ancient bathing rituals grew from the recognition that water is an elemental force that has great power to heal. In India, there are many sacred places to which people travel for thousands of miles to go and bathe in the water's sacred energy. In Pushkar, the lake is considered to be one of the holiest bodies of water, said to be made from the tears of Shiva. Each morning there is a beautiful scene that would captivate me during my time there: against a backdrop of mountains, the sun gently rises over the lake and its light begins to dance and sparkle on the surface of the water, as women in brightly coloured saris quietly enter into the vibrant blue waters to seek healing.

In this bathtime ritual, I hope you will find inspiration to add a sacred, healing dimension to your bathing routine. If you don't have the time, even just choosing one or two extra elements from this ritual will be enough to feel like you are giving some love back to yourself.

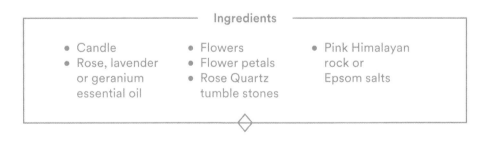

──────────── Ingredients ────────────

- Candle
- Rose, lavender or geranium essential oil
- Flowers
- Flower petals
- Rose Quartz tumble stones
- Pink Himalayan rock or Epsom salts

◇

Cleanse the bathroom

Start this ritual by cleansing the space and all your sacred ingredients in it with sage or Palo Santo wood. Even though the water itself is cleansing, the air in your bathroom can really benefit from an energetic cleanse. And, if you want some extra motivation for smudging here, then it's good to know that smudging smoke has been proven to reduce bacteria in the air by up to 94 per cent.[4] This is a quote from the study in a scientific journal in 2007: 'the ability of the smoke to purify and disinfect the air and to make the environment cleaner was maintained up to 24h in the closed room.'

Add sacred beauty to the space

After cleansing, light a candle to create a soothing ambience, and add some flowers or a plant at the end of the bath in your line of vision. This provides a beautiful focal point, allowing you to drop into a meditative state. I'll often just gaze at the flowers whilst in the bath, absorbed intimately with Mother Earth and all her natural beauty. I have this beautiful quote from Georgia O'Keeffe about flowers in my bathroom as a reminder: 'When you take a flower in your hand and really look at it, it's your world for the moment.' Maybe you have a quote that reminds you of the importance of nurturing yourself? Why not put this somewhere in your bathroom as a reminder?

For a deeper beauty bath, add some flower petals to your water. You can even dry your own flowers (rose and lavender are really good for this), then put the dried petals into a muslin bag and add this to the warm water for a deep floral infusion.

Connect to scent

To elevate your sense of smell, have a relaxing oil burning. I like to use rose and geranium oil with this specific ritual (lavender oil is also great to use here). As the aroma fills the air, I enter deeper into a relaxed state, visualizing the molecules of scent travelling up through my nose, down my chest and into my heart centre. Here, I imagine that the scent is absorbed by a delicate pink rose in the centre of my chest, slowly opening its petals to reveal a baby pink healing light. An extra touch here is to add a couple of drops of the oil into the bath and some pink Himalayan rock or Epsom salts. These salts are naturally healing and a fantastic way to help draw toxins out of the skin.

Mindfully place Rose Quartz

With this image of the pink rose firmly rooted in your heart, mindfully place some pieces of Rose Quartz around the bath. If you don't have a bath, you can simply lay the crystals around the edge of your shower tray. As I place the crystals, I imagine they are surrounding me with loving energy. I'll also add some Rose Quartz tumble stones (small polished stones) to the water, so that when bathing I'm fully immersed in a nurturing, calming, loving energy. This is the perfect energy to prepare you for a rejuvenating night of beauty sleep.

Let the deep relaxation begin

Once in the bath, I close my eyes and mindfully connect with the sense of being enveloped in water, taking a moment to express gratitude for this moment. I then imagine that the crystals surrounding me are holding me in a loving, active embrace. Feeling this embrace brings me a deep sense of calm, like I can just let go and allow myself to be supported.

End with gratitude

When you've stepped out of the bath or shower, it's important to bring this ritual to a close by expressing gratitude: for the water, the flowers, the crystals, for this time to restore yourself. I like to listen to the first sounds of the water draining, carrying away all the troubles of the day.

♥ Extra touch

When you want to add some extra Inner Beauty magic to your bathing routine, but you don't have time to do the whole ritual, you can mindfully add some small Rose Quartz chips into the bottle of bath oil or bubble bath you already use (remember to always cleanse and fill the stones with your loving intention first). This will infuse them with the calming, nurturing energy of the stone. Some of my favourite bubble baths/bath oils to use are by Neal's Yard Remedies and I sometimes like to make my own.

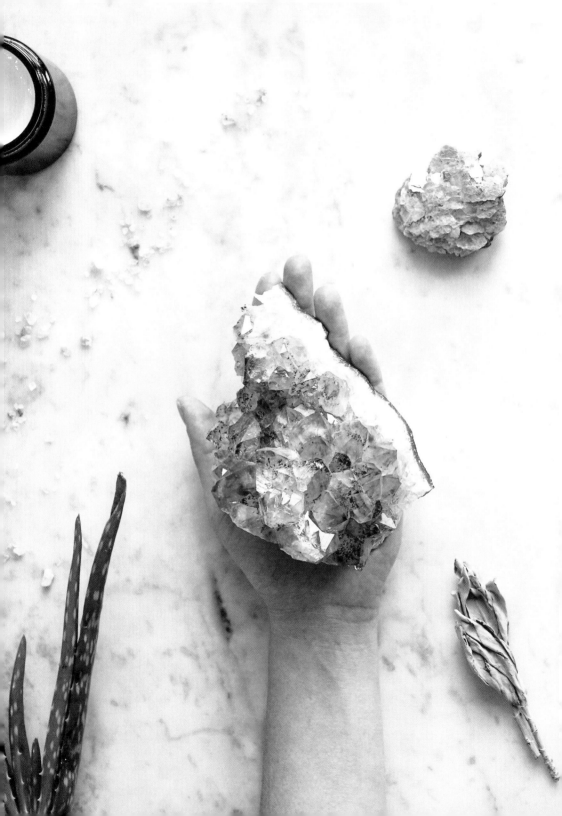

Inner Beauty Sleep Ritual

☽

'We see the beauty within and cannot say no.'
Dave Eggers, *A Heartbreaking Work of Staggering Genius*

In Kabbalah, sleep is a time when the soul leaves the body to connect with the higher spiritual realms, where it receives nourishment, rejuvenation and guidance. If we prepare ourselves in the right way, our unconscious minds will use sleep to resolve any lingering issues from the day, even bringing us insights and a sense of clarity and peace when we awaken. The Native American Blackfoot tribes believed that a butterfly (symbol of transformation) would bring us dreams in our sleep that could help us to change. They would paint a butterfly on the door of their lodges and sing lullabies inviting the butterfly spirits to come and guide their dreams. During sleep, in the words of Dave Eggers, if we prepare well, we can 'see the beauty within and cannot say no'. But without this sacred preparation, the night-time can be as exhausting as the daytime, as we struggle to sleep, or sleep lightly, or have tiring or emotional dreams. Think about what routines help you to have a sound night's sleep. What objects do you like to have in your room to bring peace?

Make your bedroom into a sanctuary for Inner Beauty

Does your bedroom make you feel calm and relaxed? There are some really simple and obvious things that you can do with an extra touch of mindfulness to turn your bedroom into an Inner Beauty sanctuary. We all know that cosy feeling of having freshly laundered linen and nicely puffed-up pillows into which you can just let your head sink deeply. Here are some other tips for you:

Declutter It really helps to take time to declutter your bedroom. I know from personal experience that bedside tables can become a dumping ground for loose change, odd buttons, random stuff, but ideally we want to keep these drawers tidy and organized as this will help our minds to relax for sleep.

Nature I recommend bringing some Nature into your bedroom. Some plants that can support Inner Beauty sleep are lavender, peace lilies and jasmine. NASA did a study in the 1980s of which indoor plants would support the purest and cleanest air for their space stations, and peace lilies were one of the best.[5]

Scent Having an oil diffuser in your bedroom can really help to promote a peaceful night's sleep too. I love to use frankincense, lavender and angelica root oils. Angelica root has been used as a healing plant for at least 2,500 years, described as a powerful cure in ancient Ayurvedic texts. It's known to protect us from negative energies, and so it's a really good ally to ensure our dreams are playgrounds of love, not fear. I usually mix angelica root with lavender, as the scent of the root on its own can be a little overwhelming.

Himalayan crystal rock salt lamps For peaceful lighting in your bedroom, Himalayan crystal rock salt lamps are wonderful Inner Beauty tools. Not only do they provide a soft, warming, orange light, but they also generate negative ions. Negative ions are what we find in abundance in forests and the sea; generally in places of Nature. Too many positive ions in the bedroom can disturb our sleep, as they reduce blood and oxygen supply to the brain, so I like having one of these lamps in my bedroom.

Crystals for the bedroom Amethyst is a perfect crystal for the bedroom. Known as a 'master healer', Amethyst, with its soothing purple tones, brings calming and peaceful energy as well as protection. You can place Amethyst on your bedside table or under your pillow. Sometimes, if I've been having challenging dreams, I'll place Amethyst tumble stones under my bed on each of the four corners, and this helps to restore protective energy to my dreamworld. Lepidolite is another great stone for the bedside table, as it connects us to emotional healing and peace. This crystal is rich in the mineral lithium, which as we know is used as a sedative, so it's no wonder that Lepidolite transmits an energy that can support our deep relaxation and sleep. Some other suggestions for crystals to pop under your pillow or on your bedside table include Moonstone, Rose Quartz and Amber, all good for helping to support sleep.

Homemade pillow/linen spray One lovely bedtime Inner Beauty tip involves a homemade pillow/linen spray. Fill a small glass spritzer bottle with water (natural, where possible), add a couple of drops of lavender essential oil and a couple of small Amethyst chippings. When you spray this on your pillow and your linens, the scent of this magical potion will help rock you gently to sleep.

Dreamcatcher A dreamcatcher is a beautiful, sacred piece of art, originally from the Ojibwe Native American tribe. It is made to resemble a spider's web, and its purpose is to filter out any bad energies or dreams, only allowing good thoughts to enter our mind and body during the night. I have one hanging behind my bed, and I like to cleanse it in the morning with some sage from time to time.

Unplug Now your bedroom is perfectly primed for your Inner Beauty, a key first step in your bedtime ritual is to unplug from the day. I know this can be particularly hard as we do almost everything on our devices. One thing I've learned recently which made me think twice was that the blue-spectrum light of our phones and computers actually limits the production of melatonin, the sleep hormone. With this in mind, it can help to switch our devices off before bedtime (even if it's only for a few minutes), especially if we are struggling to sleep well. When you decide to turn off your computer or phone, connect with the feeling that you are saying goodbye to that world for the night so that you can restore your Inner Beauty. If you really must have your device in bed, there are some great apps that are designed to change the colour of your screen to help you drift off. If you use your phone as an alarm, it can help to put it into flight mode before you go to sleep.

Cleanse for Inner Beauty sleep

Once you've unplugged, an important part of this bedtime ritual is to give yourself and your bedroom a good energetic cleanse. I normally use Palo Santo wood as it has less smoke and a softer scent. I walk around the bedroom with the wood burning, cleansing each of the four corners of any heavy energies lingering from the day and welcoming in a peaceful night's sleep. I then cleanse myself. As I wave the Palo Santo around my body, I bring to mind something I want to let go of from the day, something that I might be worried about, perhaps an uncomfortable conversation. As always, make sure the window is open. I like to stand at the window and watch the smoke travel out into the night sky, taking my troubles from the day with it.

Night-time gratitude

Once you've climbed into bed, just before you go to sleep, nestled in your fluffed-up cushions, now is the ideal time to practise gratitude. Thinking about things you are grateful for before you drift off will encourage your mind to stay connected to your heart in the Land of Nod. I have a gratitude journal which I keep on my bedside table. I write at least one thing I'm grateful for from the day just gone. I also bring to mind one thing I'm looking forward to for the following morning. For me, I really look forward to my cup of coffee and the whole ritual around it. This can also be a perfect way to connect with your partner or children, sharing with each other those things you're grateful for before you go to sleep.

Bodyscan

If you have trouble getting to sleep, this really simple technique my husband taught me from the mindfulness tradition can help take your attention away from any worries in your mind. All you have to do is bring your attention into your body. You can start from the top of your head, just noticing what sensations are there. Whatever you notice, bring a quality of acceptance and compassion. Slowly make your way down, checking in with the sensations in each part of your body. As you practise this, you'll find it easier to drop into your body and drift into a natural, peaceful sleep.

Dream journal

In the Western world, unless you are working with a dream-focussed therapist, dreams are not given anywhere near as much attention or value as in indigenous cultures. Native people use dreams to find answers to their life-problems, to communicate with their guides or Higher Self, to heal psychological wounds and even physical illness. So if you're curious about enhancing the Inner Beauty potential of your dreams, start by keeping a dream journal, writing as many details as you can remember from the night's dreams. As you start to keep track of your dreams, look out for patterns and pay attention to how your dreams make you feel – these feelings are your guide.

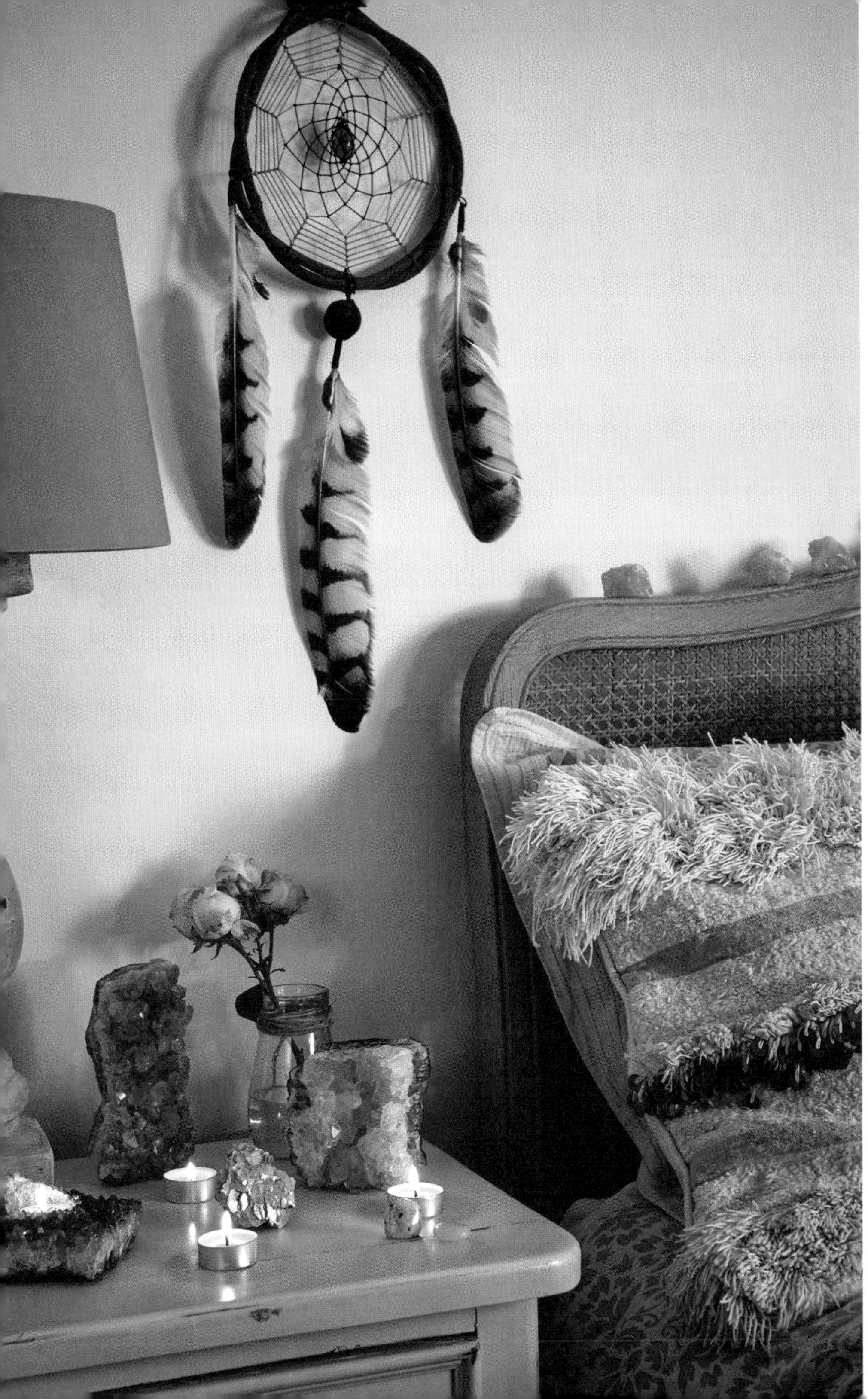

Inner Beauty on the Move

'When the wind of change
blows, some build walls,
others build windmills.'

Chinese Proverb

6

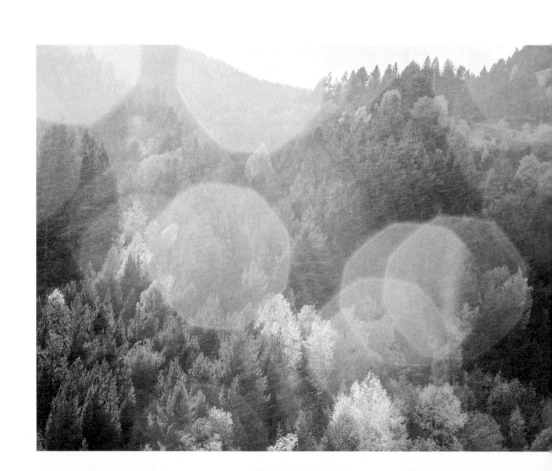

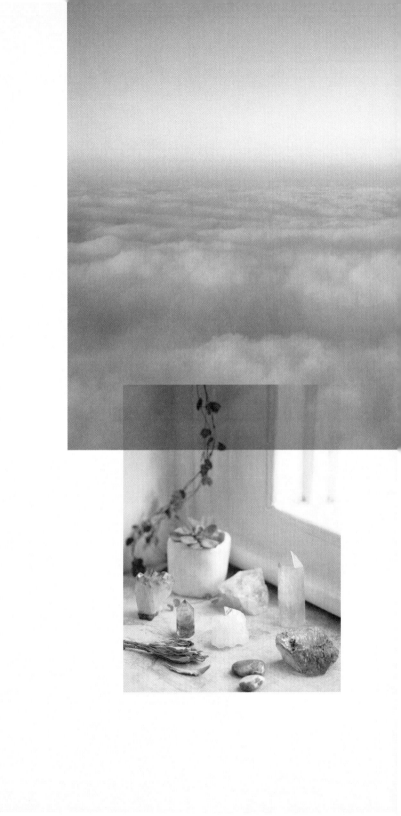

Be a Windmill,
Not a Wall

We are living in a time of rapid change. The idea of a 'job for life' seems quite old-fashioned already. We don't stay in the same relationships as often as we used to. We change homes, change cities, change countries even. Our life-path is an increasingly winding road with a dizzying number of twists and turns. With all this uncertainty, life can feel quite overwhelming. Learning how to master transitions, how to master the flow of energy as we move from one state to another, from one situation to another, is a vital life-skill in the twenty-first century. Rituals are a perfect tool to support us in this: they can be a helpful anchor, providing us with a sense of perspective, wisdom and grounding in the accelerating ebb and flow of life.

How do you feel about change? Do you cling to the old or do you chase after the new? What transitions have you had to manage in your own life – e.g. changes in family life, moving home, moving jobs, starting a new relationship – and what helped you to manage them? I've been through quite a number of transitions in my own life: since my early teens right up until the present moment, there have been several disruptions in my family unit, all steep learning curves for me. I'm not really sure I knew how to manage these transitions back then. But now, although I'm learning every single day, I've picked up along the way some wonderful methods of working with the energies of change and uncertainty. The key is remembering. Remembering Inner Beauty qualities can be a real challenge, especially when we find ourselves outside our comfort zone, and our tendency is to hide away in old habits. But, as Neale Donald Walsch says, 'Life begins at the end of your comfort zone … if you're feeling uncomfortable right now, know that the change is a beginning, not an ending.' I hope that some of the practices I share in this chapter will help you in times when you find yourself feeling uncomfortable or outside of your comfort zone, to remember your Inner Beauty when life around you seems unsteady, so that you can be a windmill and not a wall.

'Learning how to master
transitions, how to master
the flow of energy as
we move from one state
to another, from one
situation to another,
is a vital life-skill in the
twenty-first century.'

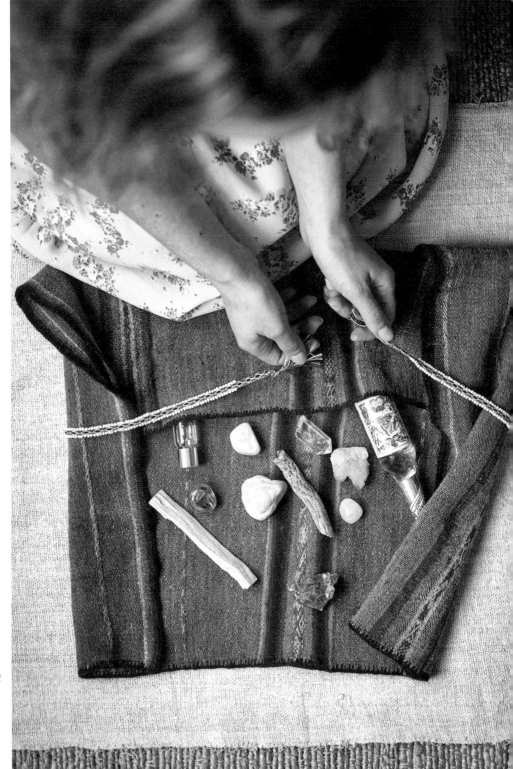

Portable
Inner Beauty

How can we stay connected to our Inner Beauty when moving from one situation to another? I have fond memories of staying with families whilst travelling around India and feeling super-inspired by the beautiful sacred spaces that these families paid such loving, daily attention to. So I decided to start setting up my own sacred space on the go. I found an antique piece of handmade Indian cloth which I'd lay out in a corner of our room, and mindfully arrange my incense, stones, singing bowl and some flowers. I'd do this in every place we stayed, no matter whether it was a simple hostel or a fancier hotel. This portable Inner Beauty temple was a precious reminder. Whenever I laid my eyes on this sacred space, I really felt that both the room and myself were being blessed by that generous energy of beauty.

There were definitely more challenging times and places when this energy was really needed. I remember arriving in the middle of the night in a very remote location after a scary tuk-tuk ride through deserted, pot-hole-lined alleys to find our room literally swarming with insects, and no one to speak to. After a restless night's sleep where we had swaddled ourselves head-to-toe in blankets to try and stop the bugs from getting us, the next morning we realized that the bugs were attracted by a small fluorescent lamp. As soon as it was turned off, they all disappeared! The room was now seriously in need of some Inner Beauty magic, and so I remember taking extra time and care to do a deep energetic cleanse and to create an especially beautiful sacred space here.

Whenever we're moving from one place to another, even if it's just catching the bus home or to work, transitions can certainly be testing. I know all too well the impact it can have on our energy when we're travelling to work on an overcrowded train: we can't get a seat, crammed in like sardines, the person next to us keeps banging us with their big, heavy bag. Transitions such as this can leave you in a foul mood for the rest of your day. Which is why, in the same way that you might carry a little make-up bag with you to touch up your outer beauty, a small bag of Inner Beauty magic can help you to touch up your goddess energy throughout the day.

In Peru, I learned from our wisdom teachers about the wonderful Andean tradition of the *mesa*: a sacred bundle that people carry around with them wherever they go. These bundles were composed of a soft cloth tied up with a ribbon, and inside the bundle there could be stones or crystals from special or sacred places, special notes from people, and any other sacred items whose energy a person might want to bring around with them. This was portable Inner Beauty in its most inspirational form. And one aspect of this indigenous practice we really loved was that, whenever we visited a sacred site, we would open our bundle and allow our sacred items to be charged by the energy or spirit of that place. I'll never forget the special Winter Solstice sunrise in Isla del Sol on top of a sacred mountain, sitting amongst our group of shamans and friends, a row of mesa bundles all opened up in congregation to the rising sun, the crystals responding to the first rays with shimmering smiles as they soaked up the energy of this beautiful moment. But you don't need to be a million miles from home to find a place in Nature that is sacred to you.

Choose your vessel

Your first step is finding something to carry your Inner Beauty tools around with you. In the *mesa* tradition, the cloth used is often quite large and not really accessible for us modern girls with our already stuffed-to-the-brim handbags. Although I have my own *mesa* that I usually take with me only when I visit sacred sites, most days I like to carry a small bag with a pull-string that is just big enough to contain a couple of crystals and an essential oil. These smaller bags are similar to medicine bundles in Native American tradition and mojo bags in African–American folk tradition (they have a lovely description for these as 'prayers-in-a-bag').

SUGGESTIONS FOR INNER BEAUTY ON-THE-GO KITS:

Everyday Inner Beauty kit

This kit is a general multi-purpose kit that you can bring to work, or generally for when you're out and about during the day, supporting you to stay connected to that sense of magic in your everyday life. My suggestions for crystals to include in this kit are: Rose Quartz (for love and nurture), Clear Quartz (for energy boost, clarity of mind and focus), Amethyst (for inner peace, calming energy and protection), Smoky Quartz or petrified wood (for gentle, grounding energy). I also include some Inner Beauty scent. The ones I tend to use for this everyday kit are Rose Absolute oil, Palo Santo wood, a small bottle of Agua de Florida, or some lavender from the garden.

Travel kit

The following describes the basic tools I recommend having in your Inner Beauty bag whenever you're going away. For crystals, I recommend: Amethyst (for protecting travellers), Hematite (grounding and helps with jet-lag), Smoky Quartz (protection from negative energies). For smells, I like: orange and peppermint oils (I find these really help me with travel sickness), and a rose facial spritzer to refresh, keep my skin hydrated and bring me back to presence when I'm tired.

Most of the rituals in this book can be transformed into a little magic bag for when you're on the move. For example, if you've done an abundance ritual in the morning and you want to bring that abundant energy with you throughout the day, you can put the Citrine you used, the abundance statements you wrote, the photo of a happy memory, all in your mojo bag.

A FEW DIFFERENT WAYS TO CONNECT WITH YOUR INNER BEAUTY KIT:

Keep it close to you

It can really help, especially if you're on a potentially stressful journey, to keep your Inner Beauty bag in your pocket. Or you can take one of the stones out and place it next to the skin, holding it in your hand or sometimes I even tuck it into my bra.

Keep it simple

I appreciate that sometimes our days are super-busy as we fly around from one place to another. These kits and different ways to connect are just suggestions, and sometimes all we might need is to have one single crystal or an essential oil on us; connecting with just one Inner Beauty tool can be enough to support us in transitions. Sometimes, when I'm running from A to B with a heavy make-up kit, I'll just have a little crystal tumble stone (often a Rose Quartz) on me, and an oil (often pink lotus) that I'll smell whenever I want to reconnect or de-stress.

Set up a sacred space on the go

You can create a beautiful but simple sacred space on the go by arranging the Inner Beauty tools on your work desk or in the room you are staying in. If you work at a desk with a computer, ideally you want to set up your sacred space in your line of view but away from the computer. This can then be a beautiful break for your eyes from the screen.

Inner Beauty break

If you feel you need a mindful break from a piece of work you've been doing, or if you've just had a difficult meeting, you can use the tools in your kit to create an Inner Beauty Break. If I have Palo Santo with me, and I've had a difficult encounter or meeting, I like to give myself and the space I'm in a quick cleanse, so that I can enter into the next moment with fresh energy and presence. For times and places we can't just whip out the wood and start burning, for fear of setting off a fire alarm or just maybe looking a bit too woo-woo in front of our colleagues, a good alternative is to have a small spritzer with water and either a Snowy Quartz crystal and/or a few drops of Holy Basil oil inside. A quick spritz around yourself and the room will give things a good energetic cleanse, making you feel fresh and ready to start again. If you're feeling stressed, you can combine the scent-based cleanse with a super-simple two-step mindful meditation.

Step 1 – Acknowledge: Simply close your eyes and bring your awareness to what's going on inside you. How does your mind feel now? Is it stressed or relaxed or somewhere in between? How does your body feel right now? Does it feel tense or relaxed or somewhere in between? The simple act of acknowledging is a very grounding practice, especially when we are busy and on the move and can easily become disconnected from ourselves.

Step 2 – Accept: Now you have checked in with your inner world, see if you can let go of the part of you that is trying to fix things. You might notice this as an uncomfortable energy somewhere in your body or a subtle thought in your mind that gives you the sense that whatever you are feeling or thinking right now is somehow wrong, not enough. Just allow the energies to be as they are. Bringing the energy of acceptance overrides judging, stressed-out energies. For an extra touch, I like to place a nurturing hand on my stomach and connect with the rise and fall of my breath.

See the beauty in the everyday

Another small but powerful practice for when you are in transit involves looking for one beautiful thing in the people and places you see. When we are on the move and, especially in busy cities, passing hundreds of different, anonymous faces, our minds can tend to fall into introverted judging. To reverse this trend, a really nice, playful exercise is to look for one beautiful thing about anyone your eyes fall upon. Everyone has at least one beautiful thing. It might be their smile, their freckles, the care they've taken to dress themselves, the kind or gentle way they've interacted with someone. Whatever it is, just by noticing it we are retraining our minds-on-the-move to connect to a sense of appreciation. The same can apply to the environment we're passing through. Again, in a built-up city like London, it can be easy to feel gloomy and get introverted, especially on a rainy day, as we traipse past row after row of grey, anonymous buildings or chain stores. But there is always something beautiful to notice, whether it's the small flower growing in the crack of the pavement, the beautiful brickwork in a building, or the warm light of a lamp post reflected in a puddle before us. If you need any inspiration, listen to these wonderful words from Roald Dahl: 'And above all, watch with glittering eyes the whole world around you because the greatest secrets are always hidden in the most unlikely places. Those who don't believe in magic will never find it.'[6]

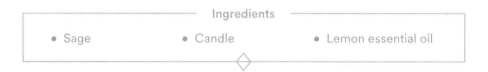

According to a recent study, the average British person moves eight times in their life, with 83 per cent finding the move very stressful.[7] I know when I've moved home in the past, I could easily feel overwhelmed by the sheer volume of stuff I'd accumulated and by the physical and practical task of packing it down, transporting it, and then unpacking it. But, in many ancient and indigenous traditions, moving home was a time for ritual, ceremony and celebration. So why not add a dash of mindfulness and a little magic into the process? As the saying goes, home is where the heart is. So if we want to make moving home into a more beautiful, life-enhancing process, then we need the right Inner Beauty tools … and a big dose of TLC.

Ingredients

• Sage   • Candle   • Lemon essential oil

◇

Say goodbye to the old house

When you've packed all your stuff up, even though you're stood there gazing at an empty shell, the memories still speak to you: the faded red-wine stain on the carpet from the party, the kids' height markings on the wall, the holes where pictures and paintings once spread joy into a space. As we say goodbye to an old home, we want to ensure we bring the good energies and memories with us. A really nice way to do this, before you close the door for the last time, is to sit in your favourite spot and light a candle. As you watch the candle, mindfully invite all those joyful, positive memories and energies that have been lived out in this space to join the next phase of the journey with you. Visualize the candle absorbing all this joy to bring into your new home. Whenever you feel ready, blow out the candle and bring it to your new home.

Inner Beauty on the Move

Deep energy cleanse your new home

To make your new space into a home sweet home, it's important, first and foremost, to give it a good physical clean. In the Feng Shui tradition, it's recommended to buy new brooms and mops and throw away the old ones, as you don't want to 'sweep in your old troubles' with the broom from your last house. As an extra touch, I add a little lemon essential oil to any water I'm using to clean (not only does it smell gorgeous but it also helps to cleanse the energy). After the physical cleanse, it's also really important to give the energy of your new home a deep cleanse too. The energetic cleanse should be done before unpacking. First, open the windows in the house, allowing the stale air and energy a way out. Then, get yourself into a peaceful, mindful space by taking a moment to close your eyes and cleanse yourself. You can use a number of different cleansing tools here: sound, Palo Santo or sage. A friend and Native American wisdom-keeper recommends sage for house cleansing as it creates more intense smoke and is more effective at covering a bigger area. When you feel ready, walk around the house with your cleansing tool of choice. Move around each room with a special focus on the corners of the rooms, as this is where stagnant or heavy energy can accumulate. As you move about, you can either repeat cleansing affirmations to yourself (such as, 'I welcome new, fresh energy into this space'), or you can visualize the old energies leaving the space along with the smoke. In each room, keep moving around with your cleansing tool until you get a deep sense that the energy of the room has been purified, and the colours are brighter, sparkling, and you feel lighter as you stand there.

Set a clear intention for your new home

Once you've cleansed the home, now is the time to get really clear on your intention. Ask yourself: 'What is my deepest wish for this home?' Take your time. This is a big move, and you want to get this right. Is this primarily a place you want to raise a family? Do you want to create a sanctuary for yourself? Or build your career? Or is this a place where you want to bring joy and laughter with friends?

Seal your intention

When you feel clear on your deepest wish for this home, now is the time to light the candle you brought from your old house. As you gaze at the smoke from the candle, imagine all the positive and joyful energies of your old place merging through the smoke with all the fresh, exciting possibilities of this new home. Allow your imagination to roam to three years from now: what wonderful experiences are you having in your home? What friends and family are you spending time with here? What feelings are arising as you imagine these special moments in your new home?

Place crystals

Moving into a new home is an opportunity to place your crystals in a way that will help to support you in your new life. Needless to say, give your crystals a good cleanse before placing them. When we moved recently, one of the things I was most excited about was adding Inner Beauty to each room by placing crystals in certain areas. So I put Rose Quartz just inside the front door so that people are greeted with loving energy when they enter.

I placed Lepidolite and Amethyst in the corners of the bedroom for peace and a good night's sleep. Apophyllite was my stone of choice for the living room: its gentle, peaceful, spiritual energy is perfect for the room where I keep my main sacred space and where my husband and I run our meditation groups. I put Fluorite and Tree Agate in the plant pots in the home and garden to encourage growth and beauty. I even placed some Rose Quartz underneath the bathtub, as we were having a new bathroom fitted. When you're placing crystals in your new home, be guided by your own intuition.

'So if we want to make moving home into a more beautiful, life-enhancing process, then we need the right Inner Beauty tools ... and a big dose of TLC.'

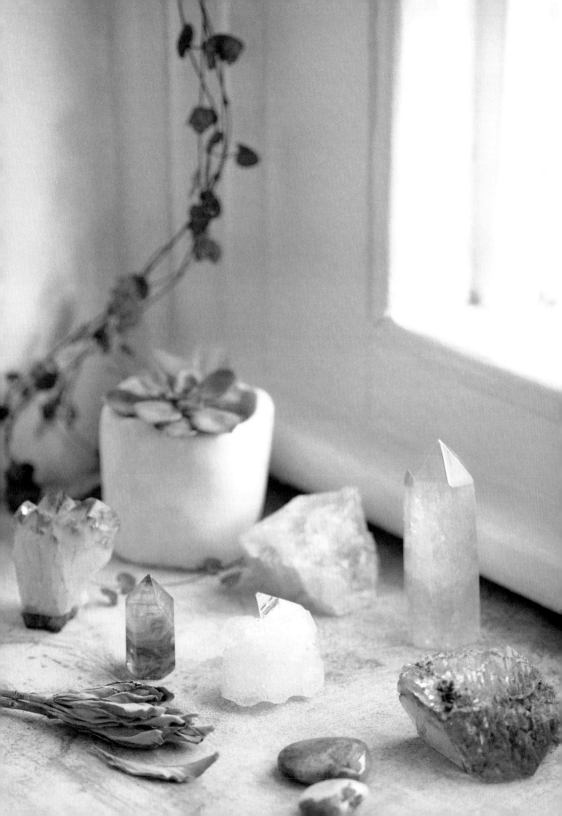

Nature Rituals

'At the fundamental level
Nature, for whatever
reason, prefers beauty.'

David Gross, physicist, Director
of the Institute of Theoretical
Physics at UC, Santa Barbara

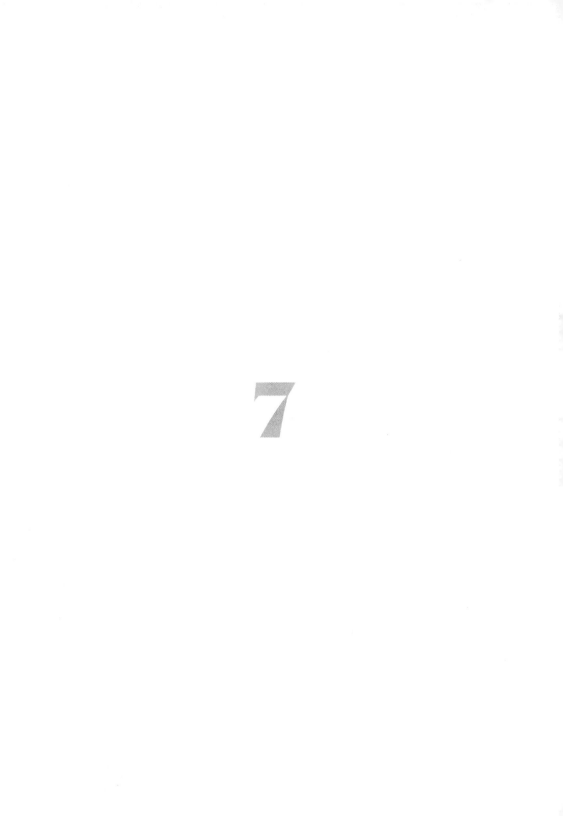

7

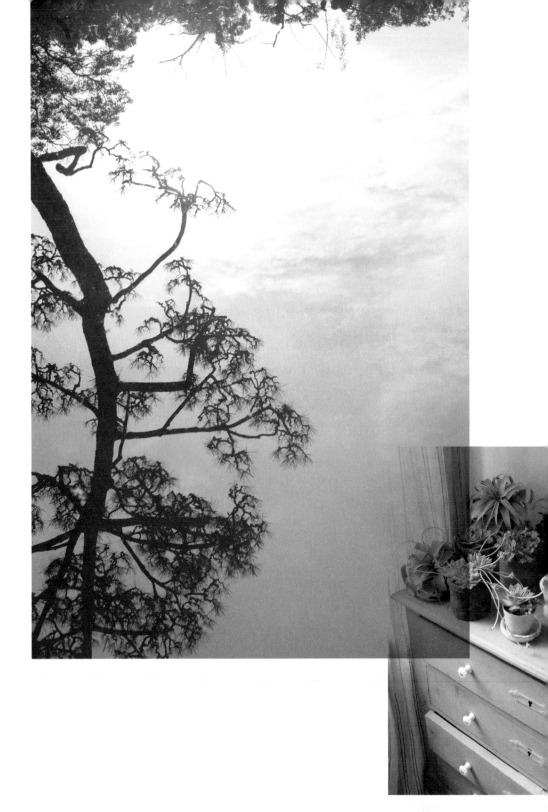

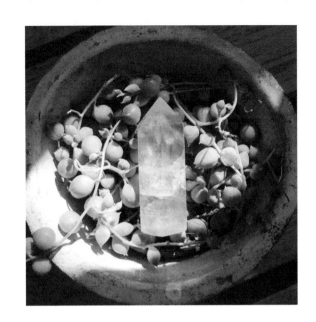

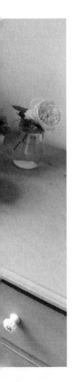

Mother Nature
is a Healer

Mother Nature is a healer. In Japan, there's a form of natural therapy called *shinrin-yoku* ('forest-bathing') where patients spend time walking through forested areas inhaling the woody scents. It has been found that, compared with people walking through urban areas, forest-bathers had lower blood pressure, lower pulse rates and lower cortisol (a stress hormone) levels. The trees are our friends!

Many shamanic and indigenous traditions have deeply honoured this healing potential of Nature. A fundamental part of their belief system is that humans aren't separate from Nature, but instead that Nature and all living things have a spirit or consciousness that will protect us if we show respect and humility – this way of relating to Nature's spirit is known as animism. In fact, because many shamanic or indigenous ways of life believe Nature has a spirit, they tend to live far more in harmony with Mother Earth than modern Western societies. For example, Inuit eskimos always take time to thank the soul of the animal they've hunted for offering itself up to them. When Maori tribespeople are digging up sweet potatoes, they will always say their thanks and blessings (*karakia*) to the spirit of the potato. I'm guessing this might seem to you quite unusual at first, thanking a potato. But, having spent some time with animist shamans and communities, I can really appreciate now how important it is to honour Nature and her gifts in this way.

Respecting the spirit of Nature is a surefire way of developing mindfulness. If you can see and know that the plants, the trees, the animals all have a consciousness just like you, you are less likely to treat them badly. So this mindfulness naturally translates into less upset for Pachamama. These words from biologist Jonas Salk sum up for me just how sacred Nature is, and how mistaken our human-centred view of life can be: 'If all the insects were to disappear from the earth, within 50 years all life on earth would end. If all human beings disappeared from the earth, within 50 years all forms of life would flourish.'

Whilst many of us urban-dwellers may not be lucky enough to live on the edge of a forest, and most readers of this book are probably not hunting seals or even pulling sweet potatoes from the ground, we can still find ways to mindfully connect with Nature, even in built-up city environments. Perhaps you have a park near you, or a canal, or just some trees. Whatever you have, the following rituals will help you to connect with Mother Nature in a deeper, more harmonious, and beautiful way.

'Respecting the spirit of Nature is a surefire way of developing mindfulness. If you can see and know that the plants, the trees, the animals all have a consciousness just like you, you are less likely to treat them badly.'

'To walk in nature is to witness a thousand miracles.'
Mary Davies

A walk in nature can be one of the best forms of therapy: and the great thing is …
it's totally free! Maybe you go for a walk to clear your head or to find inspiration.
Rebecca Solnit, author of *Wanderlust*, explains beautifully why walking can bring our
souls such benefit: 'Walking, ideally, is a state in which the mind, the body, and the
world are aligned, as though they were three … notes suddenly making a chord.'
Most of the time, though, walking is practical, a means of getting from A to B, and
many of us (myself included) often walk with our minds absorbed in our phones. But
we are blessed to have many traditions we can call upon in which walking was a
means of cultivating presence and Inner Beauty. In many Native American traditions,
walking the land is a way to get insight into and connect with the beauty and spirit
of Nature. There's a wonderful Navajo prayer, 'In Beauty May I Walk':

In beauty may I walk.
All day long may I walk.
Through the returning seasons may I walk.

Beautifully will I possess again.
Beautifully birds …
Beautifully joyful birds.

On the trail marked with pollen may I walk.
With grasshoppers about my feet may I walk.
With dew about my feet may I walk.

With beauty may I walk.
With beauty before me, may I walk.
With beauty behind me, may I walk.
With beauty above me, may I walk.
With beauty below me, may I walk.
With beauty all around me, may I walk.

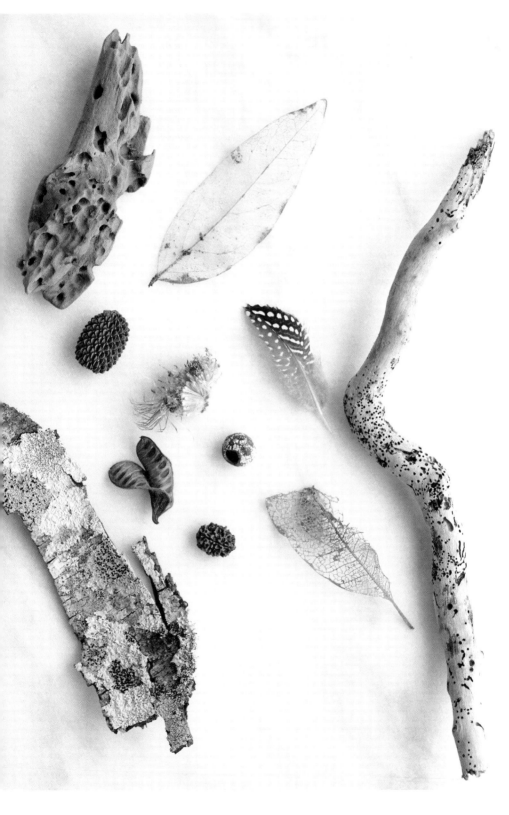

You can walk in beauty too; all it takes is adding a little mindfulness. The wonderful thing about the following ritual is that you don't need to be in an idyllic natural setting to be able to connect with Nature's beauty. The beauty of Nature is actually all around us if we look carefully. The snails that crawl out after the rainfall, the tree leaves that paint the streets in autumn, the spider's web glistening in the morning dew. So, even when you can't do the full ritual, I encourage you to take some small practices from it that appeal to you, and apply them even on your daily walk to the bus stop.

Set your intentions to release and receive

You can either set your intentions before you head off (if you have the time) or at any point whilst you are out on your walk. I have a particular tree near me where it just feels somehow like the right place to set an intention. A typical intention in shamanic traditions is to decide on something you wish to release and then something you wish to receive. For releasing, think about what attitudes, behaviours or energies you want to change or be rid of. For example, you may decide that on your walk you want to release some anger you've been holding on to about a situation that you can't really do much about. For receiving, think about what part of your life you would like some insight into. You might, for example, want to receive guidance on a particular problem you are struggling with in your work.

Choose something to release back to Mother Earth as a gift

In Q'ero indigenous wisdom, Pachamama loves to receive any heavy energy (*hucha*) that we humans create. For her, our heavy energy is like nectar, and she loves to absorb it and turn it into refined, sweet, light energy (*sami*). Inspired by this, I recommend taking some seeds on your walk which will represent your offering back to Mother Earth. These can be seeds you might already have in your cupboard, maybe pumpkin, sunflower, lavender, etc.

Spot your Inner Beauty Boosters

Whenever I walk down my street, there's a particular lavender bush that always catches my eye with its full, purple lushness creeping out onto the street, leaning out as though to greet passers-by. This bush is one of my favourite Inner Beauty Boosters. Each and every time I walk past, I stop to soak up the beautiful purple colours and gently touch the flowers to gather the scent. Even if I'm on my way to work, or in a bit of a grumpy mood in that moment, this simple connection with Nature's beauty brings me right back into my senses and gives my Inner Beauty a joyful boost. So, when you set out on your walk, look out for flowers, plants, bushes or trees that somehow call to you. Take some time to establish a connection to them. Notice what they look like, if they have a particular scent, what feelings they stir up inside you. Know that they are living beings, and that in a way they perceive you just as you perceive them. These living beings will become your allies, gracefully reminding you of the beauty at the core of your being each time you walk past. So always express your thanks to them for the gift they are sharing with you.

Release

When you are out on your walk, and you've got yourself into the spirit by connecting with some of your Inner Beauty Boosters, the next step is to find a spot that feels right for releasing. This might be a tree, a body of water, a patch of soil: any place you feel happy to pause for a moment and release into Mother Earth the thing that's been holding you back. When you've found your spot, take your seeds (or whatever releasing objects you have chosen) into your hand and bring to mind: a) the thing you want to release; b) why you want to release it; and c) how you imagine you will be once this energy is released. Now release the object into Mother Earth, by placing it in your chosen spot. Imagine Mother Earth soaking up the heavy energy like it's a sweet syrup she just loves, and instantly synthesizing it into lighter energy. This idea is taken from an Andean practice, *Saminchakuy*, where the *hucha* we are carrying is offered as a sacred gift to Pachamama so she can digest it. You may find that as you continue to walk you carry on noticing the heavy energy releasing into Mother Earth with each footstep you take. You may notice certain sensations in your feet as the *hucha* leaves your body.

Beauty Steps

If you're anything like me, you can be walking in glorious Nature and still have a mind full of to-do lists, worries and other distracting chatter. This is why I like to add a short focussed mindful part of my walk I call 'Beauty Steps', where I consciously slow my walking right down and try to make as little noise as possible, feeling my feet treading ever-so-softly on the earth below, noticing the sounds of Nature that I can now hear – as though the volume gets turned up as my mind calms. I keep this short, sometimes just a thirty-metre stretch between two trees. Of course, our thinking minds will still be wanting all of our attention, but it really helps to notice this tendency with compassion, and gently bring our awareness back to our feet and the attempt to tread delicately on the earth. In some Native American traditions, they call this the 'Fox Walk': walking so quietly that you can sneak up on an animal without disturbing it. I love this because it provides a beautiful metaphor for how we can relate to our own Inner Beauty. If we rush in, all guns blazing, looking hurriedly for the treasures within, then we will likely scare away the most beautiful parts of ourselves. If my mind is feeling particularly busy when doing my Beauty Steps, I sometimes add a little mantra: so with each delicate step, I will repeat quietly to myself: 'In beauty may I walk'.

Receiving

The wisdom that you want to receive on this walk can come at any time. If you have set your intention before heading out, an insight might hit you as soon as you step outdoors. Or the insights might come whilst getting your Inner Beauty Boost, or during your Beauty Steps. Sometimes the answer might even come later in the day or even in the week. The key is to remain open and receptive: don't try to force the answer. Remember, the best insights come when we are relaxed and open, so just be extra mindful of the thoughts and images you receive whilst on your walk. You might find yourself drawn to a particular tree, flower, plant or body of water. If you do, get close to or touch the natural thing that is calling you, close your eyes and establish a heart connection with the energy of this aspect of Mother Nature. Be open to receive. Nature can provide us with great wisdom if we let her in. You might remember the magical scene from *Alice in Wonderland* when the flowers start singing to Alice, as follows:

> You can learn a lot of things from the flowers,
> For especially in the month of June,
> There's a wealth of happiness and romance
> All in the golden afternoon

Gratitude Tree

For an extra splash of gratitude, it can be really heart-warming to finish your walk by bringing to mind things you are feeling grateful for in your life right now. I actually have a particular tree, a Gratitude Tree, that I'll sit or stand under and reflect on the things I'm grateful for, tying some ribbon or a piece of string to a branch as a testament to my heartfelt appreciation. This is a lovely way to affirm your gratitude and, as the ribbons build up on the tree, the visual beauty of this can fill your heart right up every time you see it. I can imagine this one is also really fun to do with kids.

'The wonderful thing about the Mindful Beauty Walk Ritual is that you don't need to be in an idyllic natural setting to be able to connect with Nature's beauty. The beauty of Nature is actually all around us if we look carefully. The snails that crawl out after the rainfall, the tree leaves that paint the streets in autumn, the spider's web glistening in the morning dew.'

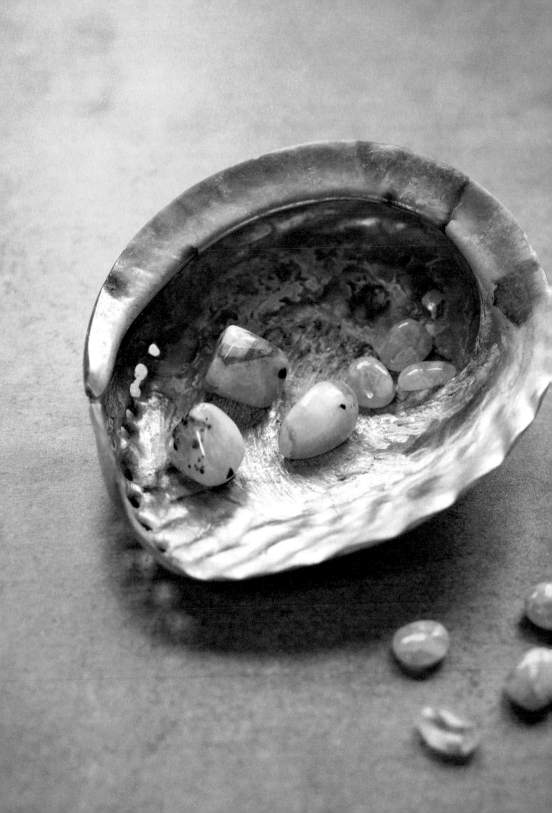

Moon Rituals

'Let the waters settle and you will see the moon
and the stars mirrored in your own being.'

Rumi

Where Nature is Mother, the Moon is Grandmother. The Moon has many magical and mysterious effects on Nature, from the rise and fall of the tides, to influencing mating patterns in various animals and affecting (some would say) women's menstrual cycles. (The word 'menstrual' comes from the Greek *menus*, meaning 'moon' and 'power'.) Have you ever noticed a change in how you feel or act then looked into the night sky and seen the Full Moon? I find it reassuring that my body is intimately connected to the Moon. In cultures where the power of the Moon in Nature was recognized, certain rituals would be held. Mothers in the Baganda tribe of central Africa would bathe their newborn children by the light of the Full Moon to help them grow healthy and strong. In Inka wisdom, Mama Killa (the goddess of the Moon) is a protector of women, and her home, at 'Isla de la Luna' in Lake Titicaca, Bolivia, is a sacred place where women gather for ceremonies. As the Moon represents the divine feminine energy, connecting to her cycles through ritual and mindfulness allows us to replenish our own divine feminine energy. Through our connection to the Moon, we can get perspective on the challenges of being a modern woman, trying to achieve a healthy work–life balance. The Moon teaches us balance.

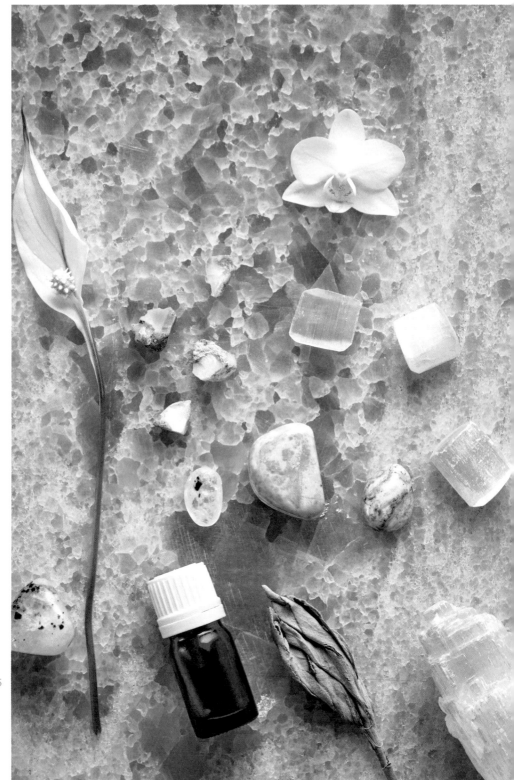

The New Moon is the day each month when the Moon is not visible from the Earth. This day has been celebrated in many different and beautiful ways around the world, but the common thread is that the Moon is full of promise and potential for growth as she begins her monthly journey from darkness to light. This is a perfect time for fresh starts, for setting intentions and manifesting. There is a beautiful and growing international tradition of women gathering together on the New Moon each month. As this is a time for manifesting, it's a perfect opportunity to gather your girlfriends together, to check in and share with each other on a deeper heart-level, and to support each other in your hopes and dreams.

In today's busy and fast-paced world it can be all too easy for our friendships to reduce to instant messages and social media interactions which rarely feel deep and meaningful. I know for myself even phone conversations I have can often feel squeezed into short time-frames as one person is going out of signal or the other just arriving at their gym class. These short bursts of interaction, lovely as they are, don't necessarily give us a safe space to chat about the deeper things that we need to feel supported in. This is why it's so important for me to create a space where my girlfriends and I can be present and vulnerable with each other. I recently discovered an amazing Harvard study which showed that not having close relationships with other women is as bad for your health as being overweight or smoking cigarettes![8] I know it can be difficult to get people together on a monthly basis, but even if you connect in this way every now and again, your heart will feel full and your relationships will feel deeper. I really hope the tools in the following ritual inspire you in gathering your girlfriends together to celebrate and cultivate our goddess energy.

Ingredients

- Suggestions for the sacred space: Selenite, Opal, or Larimar stones
- Paper and pens
- Jasmine or pink lotus oil
- Plants – for example orchids or peace lilies
- Flower petals
- Tea lights
- Ribbon or string
- Extra touch: Rainbow Moonstone

Create the group

The first step here is to decide who you would like to invite to this special gathering. This doesn't need to be a big group; if it's just two or three goddesses together, that's more than plenty, but you can gather as many as you feel comfortable with. When you have chosen your group, a fun way to organize the event is to set up a closed Facebook group (or WhatsApp group) with those girls. This can be your goddess platform, and you can use social media for a deeper connection, sharing things (inspirational quotes, poems, advice or perhaps something that happened that day, good or bad), and generally supporting each other in the unfolding of your Inner Beauty. As part of the invitation, decide on one Inner Beauty Quality that will be the theme for that month, and invite your girlfriends to bring something relating to it that they might want to share. It's always a nice touch if your girlies bring their favourite Inner Beauty tools to add to the space.

Prepare a space fit for goddesses

Once you've given the room a good energetic cleanse, make the space feel and look beautiful by lighting candles, laying cushions and blankets on the floor in a circle and creating a goddess space in the middle. The goddess spaces I create will usually have crystals such as Selenite (named after 'Selene', Greek goddess of the Moon, with a natural moonlike luminosity), Larimar (a beautiful sky-blue goddess stone found only in the Dominican Republic) and Opal (a goddess stone connected to the element of water and energy of the Moon, bringing calm). I will also add a selection of oils (including jasmine and pink lotus oil, which are good for bringing Inner Beauty, love and nurture to goddesses), some flower petals scattered in a circle around the centrepiece, and a plant that sings out goddess energy to you (I like orchids, peace lilies and, of course, roses). I also usually have a big bag of tea lights and I hand out one of these to each girl attending.

Cleanse the group

When you invite your girlfriends into your goddess space, have one of your friends greet the others as they walk across the threshold by cleansing them front and back with some Palo Santo wood or sage. This will help the girls feel that they are entering into a special moment.

Open the circle

Once everyone is sat in a circle, ask them to close their eyes for a moment, palms open, take some deep breaths and bring their attention into their heartspace. Now gently walk around the circle and put one drop of your chosen essential oil into one palm of each of their hands. Have your girlfriends cup their hands over their noses and take a nice deep breath. When they open their eyes, you can now open the circle using sound. You could simply play a beautiful song to open hearts, but if you have any sacred sound instruments such as singing bowls you can use these as well.

Inner light

Whoever is holding the space now lights a candle (ideally, you want a candle-holder with a handle to make this process easier), and passes it to the person next to them so they can light their tea light with it. This carries on around the circle until the person holding the space has the candle back and lights their own tea light. This beautiful but simple part of the ritual signifies the goddess collective making an intention to light up each other's inner light.

New Moon talk

It can be really nice at this point for you or someone in the group to share the astrological significance of this particular New Moon. Don't worry, you don't need to be an expert; I'm definitely not! Google is our friend here. One website I really love for this kind of information is Mystic Mamma (www.mysticmamma.com).

Blessing and Intention

Now is the time for everyone to check in. Ask each person to take some time to write down one way in which they would like to manifest the chosen Inner Beauty Quality in the following month – their 'Inner Beauty Intention'. For example, if the chosen quality was patience, they might set an intention to practise patience with a person or situation that tends to frustrate them. When everyone is ready, each person can take turns to share one thing they are grateful for from the last month, followed by their 'Inner Beauty Intention'. After sharing, the pieces of paper can be rolled into scrolls and tied up with a nice piece of ribbon or string and then placed in the plant, as the plant will support the growth of the group's intentions.

Seal intention

With the plant filled with all these wonderful Inner Beauty Intentions, ask everyone to close their eyes, and the person holding the space can read something out they want to share: it could be a quote, a poem, a verse of a song, or any words that come from the heart.

Heart sharing

Now the space is just open for people to share anything they might have brought with them, or any thoughts they might have on the Inner Beauty theme. Maybe they have a poem or a story they want to share. It could be an example of the Inner Beauty Quality in action. Most importantly, if anyone has something they want to share about something they've been struggling with, this can be a nice time to open the space for the possibility of vulnerability.

Close the circle

After sharing, it's time to close your circle. A nice way to do this is to get everyone to hold hands, close their eyes, and the person holding the space just gives thanks, thanking the girls for coming, for sharing, for their friendship, and finish by affirming that the group will continue to support each other as much as they can.

♥ Extra touch

A really nice extra touch here is to have a bowl of Rainbow Moonstone tumble stones in the centrepiece, and hand one out to each girl at the end of the ceremony, as a beautiful reminder of the support of their goddesses.

Sisterhood by Skype

Many of us these days have close girlfriends who live in different cities or countries. If you can't get people together in person, or if there are some special people you want to join the group who live elsewhere, you can do this circle by Skype.

Full Moon Ritual

●●●

The Full Moon is a time for completion, harvest and reflection. As a cycle of growth and glow comes to an end, this is a great time to take stock, gather what we have cultivated, let go of anything that doesn't serve us and give nourishment back to our inner goddess. I love celebrating the Full Moon, it reminds me that there are times for growth and times for retreat, times for manifesting and times to let things settle. For this ritual you'll create a bathing infusion.

Ingredients

- Cup of either fresh or dried rose petals, lavender, or camomile
- Rose Quartz tumble stone
- Small muslin bag
- Blue lotus oil (for goddess rejuvenation and insight) and/or jasmine oil
- Bowl
- Couple of Rainbow Moonstone tumble stones
- Cup of pink Himalayan rock salt

◇

Cleanse

It can be lovely to sit by a window where you can see the Full Moon or, if the weather permits, sit outside. Get yourself into a nice, peaceful, connected state by cleansing yourself, your Full Moon kit and the space you are in.

Connect with Grandmother Moon

If you can see the Moon, take a few moments to really gaze at its light. There is a beautiful ancient yoga tradition called *trataka* which involves gazing at an object such as a candle or the Moon to develop clarity and insight. Let the bright, clear light of the Moon still your mind, and when you feel ready, close your eyes and allow the image of the Moon to arise in your mind. Rumi says, 'Let the waters settle and you will see the Moon and the stars mirrored in your own being.' Allow your inner self to be absorbed by this beautiful goddess lunar energy. Notice how it makes you feel – perhaps calmer, or perhaps you have a sense of being held or of being bathed in love.

Reflect and let go

Now it's time to give yourself a precious moment of reflection. First, bring to mind one time in the last month when you felt your inner light got clouded over, when perhaps you didn't shine as brightly as you'd hoped. Maybe you were lacking in confidence, maybe you reacted with anger or impatience to a person or situation (or even to yourself); maybe you were worried about things that were out of your control. When you have this in mind, light a candle, look at the flame, take a deep breath in and as you breathe out imagine the flickering flame burning away these inner clouds.

Harvest

Now you've cleared the inner clouds, it's time to harvest the good crops you've grown over the last month. Bring to mind any shining moments from that time when you felt proud of yourself. It could be an important task you completed in work, an act of kindness you gave to someone (including yourself), or a wonderful moment shared with family or friends. As you bring each of these moments to mind, watch as they fill your heart with warmth and contentment. Allow yourself to enjoy this sense of completion and fulfilment.

Prepare your Moon bathing infusion

Fill the bowl with Himalayan rock salt. Mix in the petals and leave on a windowsill that catches the moonlight or outside if it's a dry evening. The salt crystals will harvest the Moon's energy. Leave the Rose Quartz and Moonstone there too, to bathe in the Moon's light.

Close with gratitude

Bring this part of the ritual to a close by thanking the Moon for the light she is sharing with your Inner Beauty tools. When you collect these tools in the morning, take another mindful moment, smell the petals and give thanks to the Moon again, whose light you may still be able to see in the sky.

Moon bath

Now it's time to give yourself a treat. Place the salt and petal infusion into your muslin bag with the Rose Quartz to infuse with extra love. At any time during this day or night, run a hot bath and add your moon-infusion bag to the water, along

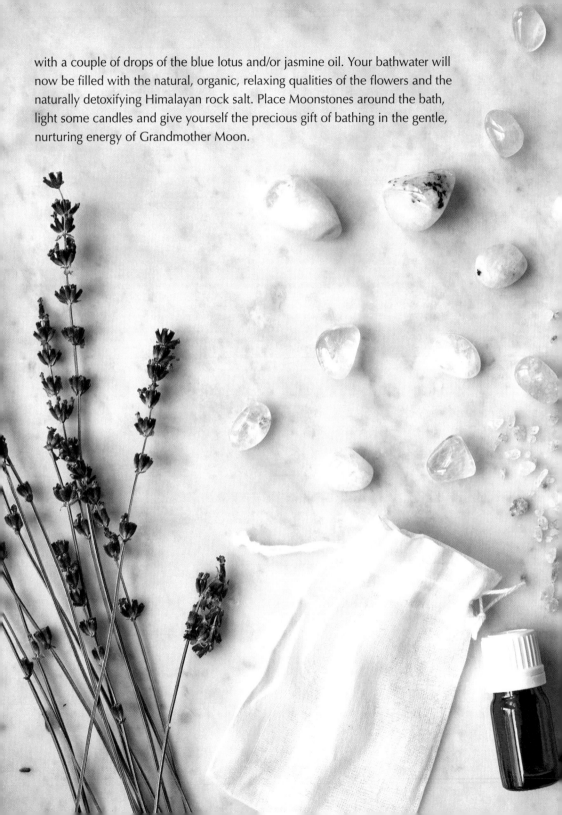

with a couple of drops of the blue lotus and/or jasmine oil. Your bathwater will now be filled with the natural, organic, relaxing qualities of the flowers and the naturally detoxifying Himalayan rock salt. Place Moonstones around the bath, light some candles and give yourself the precious gift of bathing in the gentle, nurturing energy of Grandmother Moon.

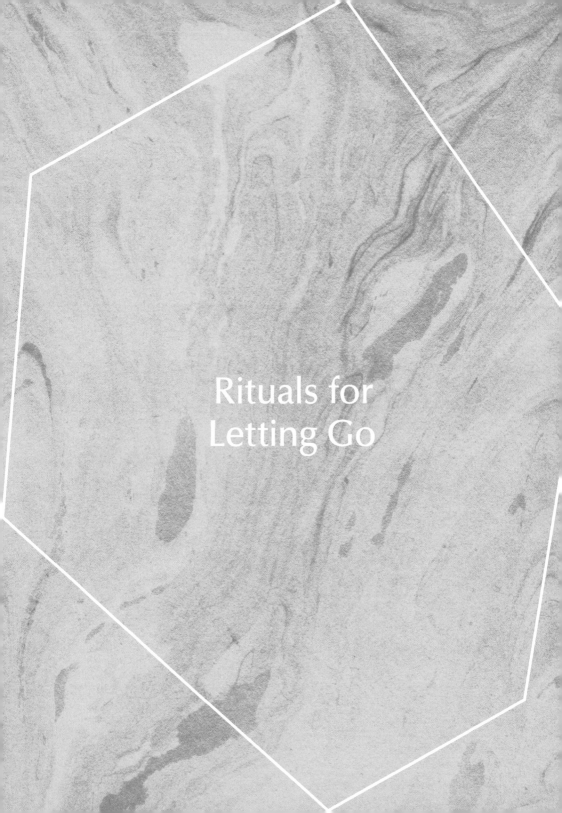

Rituals for
Letting Go

8

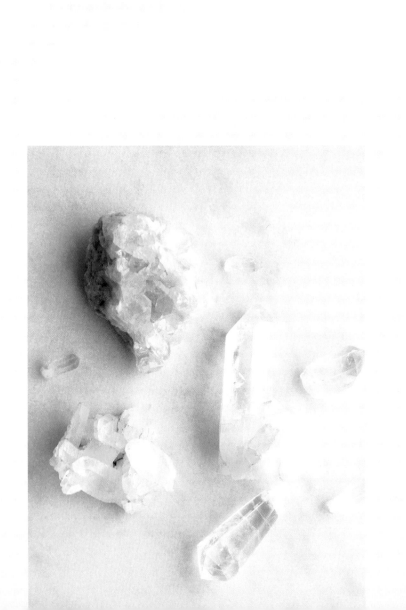

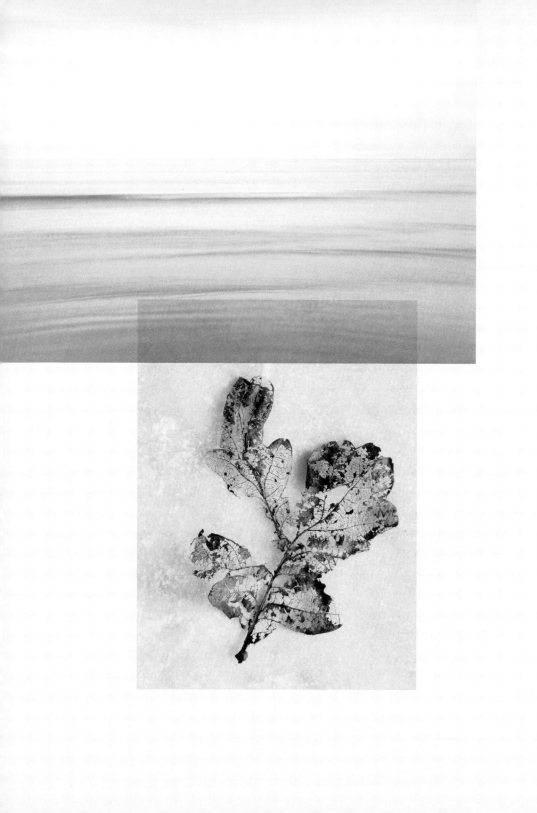

Letting Go
Makes You Lighter

Have you ever noticed how a baby instinctively grips your finger when you put it in their hand, even when they're asleep? Grasping on to things can be helpful: we could never put our lipstick on without this ability! But holding on to things emotionally can weigh us down, literally. In one study, two groups of people were asked to do a standing jump and the height of their jumps was measured.[9] One group was asked to write about times they forgave people before jumping and the other was asked to write about grudges they still held on to. The ones who focussed on moments of forgiveness before jumping actually jumped higher than those focussed on grudges. Letting go makes us lighter, but it can be one of the hardest things to do. Our minds grasp on to hopes and expectations in the same instinctive way the baby grasps a finger. When things don't go our way, the reflex to grasp remains.

Of course, letting go is not always what we want or need. When someone close to us passes away, often we want to treasure their memory. This is why so many wonderful rituals have developed around the world to help us remember our loved ones and ancestors. And letting go does not mean brushing our feelings under the carpet. Feeling is not failing. We all experience challenging emotions in our lives; sometimes even over seemingly insignificant things. But if we are stuck in the past, if our hearts stay locked down in bitterness, resentment or grief, then we can't shine our unique light into the world. Like a snake shedding its skin, when we learn to let go we can dance through this life with more freedom, lightness and grace. In the following rituals, I hope you find the courage to let go of those things, patterns and emotions that aren't serving you any more. Please do take good care of yourself too. For some difficult events in our lives we may need professional help to process and let go. I know my husband sees a lot of people in his therapy practice who have been hurt very badly, and in these cases letting go is a careful, gradual and deep process.

'If we are stuck in the past, if our hearts stay locked down in bitterness, resentment or grief, then we can't shine our unique light into the world.'

**'Forgiveness is the fragrance that the violet sheds
on the heel that has crushed it.'**
Mark Twain

Forgiveness is the ultimate act of love. Like the violet from the beautiful Mark Twain quote above, if we could respond to challenging encounters with love and not anger, then the world would simply be a more beautiful place. But of course, we can't always be violets. We are spiritual beings having a human experience, as Pierre Teilhard de Chardin wrote, and this means our delicate hearts can close up when someone hurts us, and our essence can get hidden from view. As I'm writing this chapter, I recognize that I have a lot of learning still to do in this area. As much as the spiritual pixie inside my heart knows that forgiveness is the right thing to do when I've been hurt, my human Nature can still react with the full range of emotions: anger, resentment, blame, shame, guilt. I'm learning little by little that it's important to be real about these reactions, but not to feed them. When I find myself feeding these emotions, that is when I make myself suffer.

Wayne Dyer compares resentment to being like a snakebite: it's not the bite that kills, but the venom that keeps circulating around the bloodstream. Can you recognize this process in yourself? Do you sometimes find that a negative comment or a challenging interaction can continue to affect your thoughts and feelings long after the original incident? Science is demonstrating more and more how bitterness and resentment can have a negative impact on our physical health if we allow these tainted thoughts and feelings to keep circulating around our systems. Studies show that extended feelings of anger, bitterness or resentment can affect our immune system, our organ function and our metabolism. Each time we replay in our minds the original event that offended us, the stress hormone cortisol is released into our bloodstream. I can relate to this personally. Living with Crohn's, I've definitely found that, at times in my life when I've felt hurt or betrayed, the thoughts and emotions that run around my system can end up manifesting as physical symptoms such as inflammation and pain in my stomach. On the plus side, forgiveness heals on the physical level as well as the emotional: when we make the choice to forgive, our stress levels decrease, as does our cholesterol and blood pressure, whilst our sleep and immune system functioning improves too.

If we're ever struggling to believe that we can forgive and move on, there are some awe-inspiring examples of forgiveness in human history we can remind ourselves of. Nelson Mandela's willingness to forgive after twenty-seven years in prison was the key to the end of apartheid: he summed up his thoughts in a speech given to a rally shortly after his release: 'We … need to forgive each other, because when you intend to forgive, you heal part of the pain, but when you forgive you heal completely.'

It is important to realize that forgiving does not mean forgetting. To forgive is to release *yourself* from suffering. We can do this, and at the same time hold someone to account for their actions.

The following ritual can be helpful for those times when you've had a disagreement with somebody, when you feel somebody's behaved badly towards you or you've been let down in your personal or work life, or maybe you feel you've let yourself down (the ritual applies to self-forgiveness as much as forgiving others). Whatever it is, whether it's a recent event or an older memory, the important thing is that you find yourself suffering as a result. The feelings of resentment, guilt, blame or shame are preventing your Inner Beauty from shining, and you are ready now to start letting go. Remember, forgiveness is a process, and whilst it might come easier on some days than others, we shouldn't beat ourselves up if we find patterns of resentment and blame being triggered in ourselves. The next day will always be another opportunity for us to open our hearts once again.

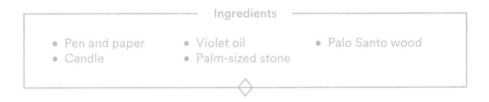

Ingredients

- Pen and paper
- Candle
- Violet oil
- Palm-sized stone
- Palo Santo wood

Cleanse

I like to use Palo Santo wood as an opening cleanse here, but you can use whatever smudging tools you want. When we move the Palo Santo around our bodies and our Inner Beauty tools and the heavenly scent drifts up through our nose, it gives a signal to our head and our heart that we're preparing to release something. As always, make sure doors and windows are open so the heavy energies can escape.

Choose one incident to forgive

It's important to get clear at the start about one specific incident that you want to forgive. We've all had some events that have continued to upset us, ranging from minor disagreements to major life events. You should begin this practice by choosing one situation that is less severe in terms of the pain it is causing you. You can often trust your mind and body here, as they will let you know if you are ready to deal with a situation. Bring to mind the incident and the person involved. If you feel any anxiety or discomfort in your body as you bring this incident to mind, take some nice, long, deep breaths.

Prepare the space

In this ritual, you'll need some violet oil, a candle and a large palm-sized stone. This could be a stone from your garden, your local park or a beach. It needs to have some weight to it. Have this stone in front of you, and then place the candle behind it and light it. As you light the candle, know that the flame represents the light of your Inner Beauty, and the heavy object represents the resentments that are weighing you down and blocking your light.

Recognize the venom

Take a piece of paper and write down three specific ways in which that original situation is still affecting you. It can help to split these three ways into the three different parts of us that tend to be affected and that interact with each other: thoughts, feelings and behaviours. Here are some examples:

Thoughts: Judging or blaming thoughts: *'I am right, and you are wrong'*; judging the person not the situation: *'X is a bad person, a nasty person.'* It might be you have the same thoughts going round and round like a washing machine driving you mad.

Feelings: Anger, resentment, upset, loneliness. Remember, feelings are never right or wrong; they just are. So try not to judge here. Be as honest as you can.

Behaviours: Avoiding situations/people, sleep affected, struggling to concentrate at work, not being present.

Now you've written down these three ways you are affected by the venom, choose a number on a scale from one to ten (with ten being the most painful and one the least) representing how much pain you've been feeling in relation to the original snakebite. Write this down on the piece of paper. This scaling question simply gives you a way to identify where you are at in terms of the need to forgive.

Hold the weight

Place the piece of paper in the palm of your hand and place the stone on top of it. Hold your hand with the stone straight out in front of you. Try to hold it there for one minute (don't worry if you find this difficult, that is the point!). Close your eyes and bring your total mindful awareness to the sensation of the weight of the stone in your hand. Really connect with this sense of weight. Notice if you can feel any sensations in your wrist and forearm relating to this weight. Maybe further up your arm and into your shoulder, and your neck too. You may feel your arm wants to drop. See how it feels to move this arm slowly up and down. Does this feel painful? Now you're really feeling the weight of this stone, bring to mind how the resentments you carry around with you might be weighing you down emotionally.

Rediscover your lightness

Now, allow the arm holding the stone to drop a little, and bring your other arm up. Bring your total mindful awareness to the feeling of lightness in this arm and hand. What can you notice differently here? Can you notice any differences in flexibility and movement? Is there less strain on your arm, shoulder or neck? Once you have connected to this sense of lightness, you can rest this arm too, and then ask yourself the following questions, allowing your imagination to explore the answers for you:

What would be the best possible outcome if you could fully forgive in this case?

> How would your thoughts be different?
> How would your feelings be different?
> How might you act differently with this sense of lightness?

Intend to forgive

If you feel ready, now is the time you can set your intention to release the weight of all this resentment that's been affecting you in relation to this person and this situation. You might want to say to yourself: 'I am ready to forgive.' As soon as you have declared your intention, open your eyes, place the stone behind the candle, then rip up the piece of paper and place these pieces under the stone. Give the stone and yourself another quick cleanse with your Palo Santo stick. Now, gaze at the candle's flame and take a moment to connect with the feeling of lightness you are hopefully now experiencing. As you continue to gaze at the candle's light, you might want to think of a small gesture through which you could express your forgiveness to the person or people you've been hurt by. If you are finding this difficult, that's fine, but you might simply want to have a moment of compassion for this person. Know that this person – including yourself – was once a baby, born into this world innocent and vulnerable with a pure and shining light. What kind of wounds might this person have experienced in their life that could have blocked this light and influenced how they responded to you?

Connect to your heart

Now add a couple of drops of the violet oil into the palms of your hand. Violet oil is known to help with letting go. Take a deep inhale, and as you breathe in feel the violet notes opening up your heart as any lingering tensions are dissolved. Remember that forgiveness is the fragrance the violet sheds on the heel that has crushed it, and that as you truly forgive you are allowing your own Inner Beauty to shine.

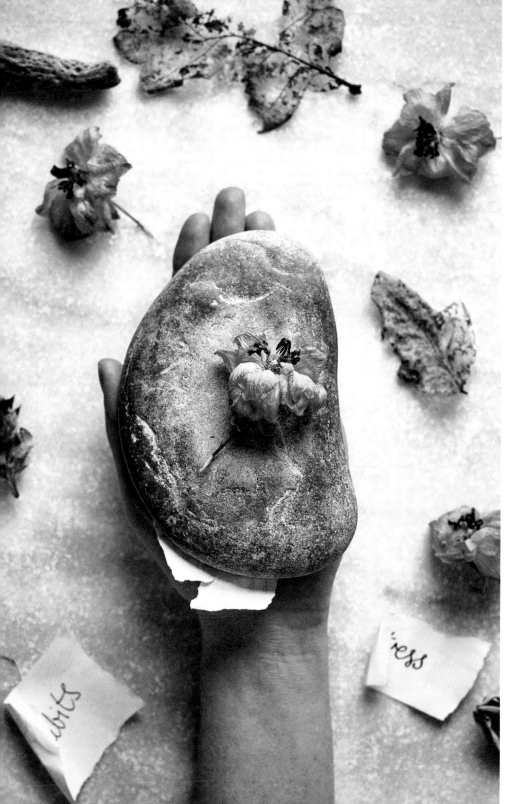

Rituals for Letting Go

Feel gratitude for the lesson

To move forward on the path of forgiveness, it really helps to finish this ritual by cultivating a space of gratitude. This might mean taking a moment to think about one lesson that this situation has taught you. Maybe there is one Inner Beauty quality that is being called forth. This quality might be empathy or compassion for the other person, or it might be humility as you let go of the need to be right. If you know the person, you can use this moment to think of one quality you can sometimes appreciate in them. Maybe they are sometimes patient or generous, or maybe they made you laugh, even if it was just one instance.

Forgiveness Reminders

Forgiveness is not something we do once and then miraculously never hold on to grudges again. It's a practice, and a quality, that we need to keep reminding ourselves of. I have a specific area in my garden that represents the main heart qualities, and in this space I have a bleeding heart plant. This plant is known to represent forgiveness and the peace we feel when we choose to release ourselves from resentment. I also have a violet-scented candle which I like to have burning whenever I feel a need to reconnect to the energies of forgiveness. Finally, I have the wonderful Hawaiian forgiveness prayer, called *Ho'oponopono*, on my wall. This prayer consists of four simple yet powerful statements: 'I'm sorry. Please forgive me. Thank you. I love you.'

'Wayne Dyer compares resentment to being like a snakebite: it's not the bite that kills, but the venom that keeps circulating around the bloodstream.'

'And the beauty of a woman, with passing years only grows!'
Audrey Hepburn

At the beginning of my make-up career, I worked with lots of fresh-faced models, their beautiful skin providing a smooth and generous canvas for my work. At that time, these girls were not much younger than me. As I got older though, the models I worked with stayed the same age. So, putting my own make-up on in the morning as I prepared for a job, my judgements about my own ageing were heightened as I'd notice the wrinkles around my eyes and the age spots changing the tone of my skin. Of course, you don't need to be a make-up artist to have these insecurities or judgements. Most of us live in societies that are clearly 'anti-ageing'. If you've got wrinkles, get botox. If you want fuller lips, collagen is your cure.

Don't get me wrong. Of course I love looking after my skin, using lots of yummy lotions and potions. But Inner Beauty is not possible until we let go of this idea that the only way to be beautiful is for us to look young. Beauty is more than skin deep, and the inescapable fact that our appearance changes as we grow older provides a perfect opportunity for us to cultivate certain Inner Beauty qualities. Amazingly, researchers at Yale University recently found that people who have a more positive attitude to ageing actually live longer than those who have a negative attitude! The following ritual is a simple practice to help you embrace ageing.

Before you begin, have a think about the following reflective questions. What fears do you personally hold about growing older? Are there any older people in your life or in the public eye who you feel are role models for how to age gracefully? What is it about these people and their relationship to ageing that you appreciate?

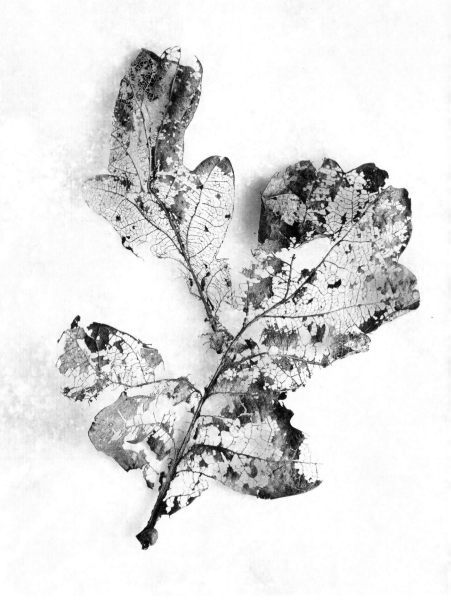

Add 'wabi-sabi' to your beauty routine

The time when we become most conscious of ageing can be during our beauty routines. So the first step towards embracing ageing is weaving in a touch of wabi-sabi here. Find an object that represents to you the wabi-sabi concept of 'beauty within the imperfections', and place this object next to your mirror, in your bathroom, on your dressing table, or wherever you tend to do your beauty routine. A few suggestions of objects that can work really well here include: an autumn leaf, a piece of driftwood, a broken crystal (many customers of The Colourful Dot ask me what to do with their crystals that have broken, and this is a perfect solution), a chipped shell, a vintage vase.

Become mindful of your self-talk

We all have that critical self-talk, especially when it comes to noticing the changing appearance of our skin and features as we get older. This self-talk is such an automatic habit that we may not even notice ourselves doing it. The more we can become mindful of this, the more chance we have of being free from it. Start to pay more attention to this negative self-talk about ageing. Whenever you catch yourself zooming in on your crow's feet, wrinkles around your mouth, or any other signs of ageing, bring your gaze instantly to the wabi-sabi object. As you're gazing at your object, see if you can gently let go of the part of you that is holding on to what was, making space to love what is. There will of course be an inevitable sense of sadness at the changes in our appearance as we age, in the same way that we experience loss at the flower losing its bloom (Ram Dass). But, over time, this practice will help you to see that there can be a beauty in your ageing, too.

Self-appreciation

As we practise letting go of our attachments to a younger version of ourselves, this frees us up to appreciate ourselves as we are right now. There are three ways I love to do this.

One is simply to appreciate the Inner Beauty benefits of being older. As they say, with age comes wisdom. Maybe you feel wiser? More confident in your own skin? More patient? Have a think now about what Inner Beauty qualities have developed for you as you've got older. Bring these to mind whenever you catch yourself in negative mind-chatter about your ageing.

The second way is to appreciate the outer beauty of your ageing self. In the same way that we can find beauty in a vintage dress or handbag, or the peeling paint on an antique piece of furniture, so too can we find the beauty in our ageing skin. When you look in the mirror, find an ageing part of yourself that you've judged. Now, as you look at this part of yourself, connect with that same appreciation you have for your vintage things and allow this appreciation to grow for your ageing self. Of course, this probably won't come easy at first. But over time this practice can really transform your capacity for self-love and, as we all know, when we can love ourselves just as we are, we are able to love others far more easily.

The third practice is simply to look into a mirror, gaze deep into your eyes and feel a connection to the ageless, timeless part of your being. Enjoy these windows to your soul. I have these beautiful words in a frame next to my bathroom mirror as a reminder of this ageless beauty:

> Beauty is life when life unveils her holy face.
> But you are life and you are the veil.
> Beauty is eternity gazing at itself in a mirror.
> But you are eternity and you are the mirror.
>
> Kahlil Gibran

'People are like stained-glass windows. They sparkle and shine when the sun is out, but when the darkness sets in, their true beauty is revealed only if there is a light from within.'
Elisabeth Kübler-Ross

Without darkness, we could never know light. Without loss, we could never appreciate life and love. As the famous lines from Alfred Lord Tennyson go: 'Tis better to have loved and lost than never to have loved at all.' We have all loved in our lives. And so we have all suffered loss in one form or another. From losing a favourite teddy bear when we were young, losing a job, a dream or a relationship, to losing someone we love, loss comes in many different shapes and sizes, as do our reactions to it. As a therapist, my husband works a lot with loss, especially with terminal illness or bereavement, and he is constantly amazed by the incredible variety of human responses to loss. Some people can move on from a loss quite quickly, whilst others can be more deeply affected.

Over the last two years, I've experienced a series of losses myself, moving through a repeating cycle of trying to get pregnant, being pregnant, and then losing the baby. It's a strange twist of fate that my most recent miscarriage coincided with my writing this chapter on Letting Go. One thing I've really learned from this journey of losses is that it's so important to give time and space to your feelings, so that they can be met with love and acceptance.

In today's world, we can feel pressured to move on quickly, get back to a 'normal' routine ASAP. Rituals allow us to create a safe and timeless zone where we can fully acknowledge our thoughts and feelings; let them breathe. Rituals can also bring a sense of order and beauty to a time of turbulence and chaos.

Having said that, grief can be complicated and sometimes we may need professional help. The following ritual is not a substitute for professional support when we find ourselves really struggling with loss.

- Pen and paper
- Object to represent loss
- Candle
- Mangano Calcite stone
- Sage
- Apple or orange
- Violet oil (for loss and grief)
- Rose petals

Find the right space

It's important that the space where we choose to do this loss ritual feels safe enough for all thoughts and feelings to arise. I prefer to find a quiet space in Nature, under a tree or ideally by water. But it can equally be done indoors, as long as you are in a space where you feel safe to allow your thoughts and feelings to come to the surface.

Cleanse

As always, when you have your space ready, make sure you give yourself, your Inner Beauty tools and the space a really thorough energetic cleanse with a smudging tool or sound.

Create a sacred circle

A circle represents a soft container – Unconditional Love. I like to create a sacred circle for this ritual using flower petals. When you have mindfully created your circle, light a candle in the middle to envoke the healing potential of the space. You might like to read Rumi's poem 'Guest House' at this point, as this poem is a beautiful expression of how to dance with difficult feelings. Here's an excerpt from the poem:

> Even if they are a crowd of sorrows,
> Who violently sweep your house
> Empty of its furniture,
> Still treat each guest honourably.
> He may be clearing you out for some new delight.

Add a symbol of the loss

Now place a symbol that represents the loss inside the circle next to the candle. This might be a picture, an object, or something from Nature.

Meditation

As you gaze into the circle, put a few drops of violet oil into the palms of your hands and breathe this in. Gently close your eyes and allow your awareness to drift down into the bottom of your body, to your feet and your connection with the earth. Imagine tree-like roots extending from the bottom of your body into Mother Earth. Watch as the roots travel through layers of soil and rock, reaching right down into the very core of Mother Earth. Feel Mother Earth supporting and grounding you through these strong roots. Once you feel grounded, allow your awareness now to rise to the centre of your chest. Place your hand on your chest to open a connection to your heart centre. When you feel a connection, you can open your eyes.

Write to let go

Take a piece of paper and a pen and write down any thoughts and feelings that have been coming up for you around this loss that may not be serving you, and any dreams and hopes that you feel you're ready to let go of in relation to this loss. When this is done, place the piece of paper in the circle next to or under the symbol of the loss.

Cleanse

If indoors, first make sure the windows or doors are open. Then take some sage, giving the symbol and the piece of paper a really good cleanse. Do the same for yourself. As you cleanse yourself, imagine the heavy energies relating to the loss leaving your body and being taken away in the smoke.

Let go

This next step is ideally done in Nature. Take your piece of paper and your symbol and (if you are not already there) bring them to somewhere either by a body of water or under a tree where you can bury them. If you are by water, you can use an apple or an orange as your vessel. Place the piece of paper in the apple or orange, set the piece of paper alight, and then let the fruit float out on to the water. As you watch the vessel float away, stay quiet and connect to the sense that the heavy energies you want to let go of are being taken away by the water and its flowing, healing energy. If you're under a tree, you can simply bury the piece of paper in the earth, along with your symbol (if it's biodegradable).

We adapted this particular ritual for our first miscarriage, using elements from a beautiful Japanese ritual for lost pregnancies, called *Mizuko Kuyo* (*mizuko* means 'water-child'). We took a picture we had from our first scan and placed it in a small hole in the earth we had prepared. We then took a small leaf and dipped it in milk and placed this leaf in the earth with the picture as a way of giving the unborn baby's soul nourishment on the journey into their next life. We also planted a flower in this spot. This plant is a symbol for us of *kokoro*, the Japanese term meaning 'it is always in my heart'.

Gratitude

Now we have let go, we end the ritual by bringing our hearts back into a space of gratitude. Rumi says:

> Don't run away from grief, o soul,
> Look for the remedy inside the pain.
> Because the rose came from the thorn
> And the ruby came from a stone.

Take a moment

Gently bring to mind one thing you can find that you are grateful for through this challenging experience. It might be that you've developed empathy for other people's suffering; it might be that this loss has brought you closer together with someone; you might feel grateful for some of the beautiful memories of the person or situation that is lost; perhaps there is some kind of meaning or lesson for you, a gem hidden within your loss. I love these words from Native-American teacher Bear Heart: 'Darkness seems like something that is hard to stand up against, but light is much stronger. Just a small light dispels the darkness.'

♥ **Extra touches**

Grief is a process, not an event, and so these are a few tips I've found useful to keep reconnecting to that space of allowing and letting go:

After this ritual, I like to keep a Mangano Calcite by my side to help soothe my heart and nurture any wounds that might have opened up during this ritual.

There is nothing more soothing than standing on a bridge looking down at water flowing beneath me. I have a small bridge near my home on the River Lea, and I sometimes like to go and stand there when an old wound reappears. In these moments, I really connect to some words I love from the ancient Chinese book, the Tao Te Ching: 'The supreme good is like water, which nourishes all things without trying to. It is content with the low places that people disdain. Thus it is like the Tao.'

Another thing I've found helpful is simply to have a really good clear-out of my wardrobe. It definitely helps me to feel lighter when I take the clothes that I don't wear or that don't bring me joy any more and drop them off at a charity shop, creating space for something new.

'In today's world, we can feel pressured to move on quickly, get back to a "normal" routine ASAP. Rituals allow us to create a safe and timeless zone where we can fully acknowledge our thoughts and feelings; let them breathe.'

Celebration
Rituals

'Let us fall in love again
And scatter gold dust all over the world.
Let us become a new spring
And feel the breeze drift in heaven's scent.
Let us dress the earth in green
And like the sap of a young tree
Let the grace from within us sustain us.
Let us carve gems out of our stony hearts
And let them light our path to Love.
The glance of Love is crystal clear
And we are blessed by its light.'

Rumi

9

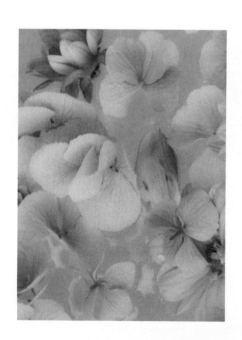

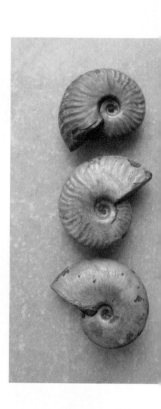

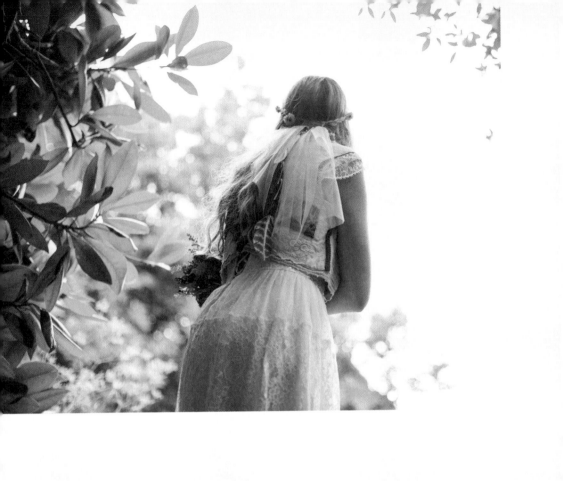

A Celebration is a Moment
Gift-Wrapped in Joy

From gentle folk-dancing around the Maypole to teeming crowds throwing fluorescent paint at each other for *Holi*, celebrations are a uniquely human way of marking special moments in our days, years and lives. Many of the celebrations we know today traditionally have a deeper spiritual significance. The idea of birthday cakes is believed to have originated in Ancient Greece, when devotees brought moon-shaped cakes adorned with candles to the temple of moon goddess Artemis; the candles symbolizing the glow of the moon. Nowadays, many celebrations tend to be less focussed on our inner connection to the sacred, and more on exterior values: what outfit we're going to wear, what present we might receive, which bottle of wine to bring.

I've definitely loved a good party, especially festivals, which for me are such a special time for celebrating with friends in music, dance and laughter. I met my husband at a festival too! As a make-up artist, I've been so blessed to find myself at the heart of so many wonderful celebrations, helping people to feel beautiful, whether it's an intimate sixtieth birthday party or a big and elaborate wedding. But, as I've wandered deeper down my spiritual path, I've started to weave more

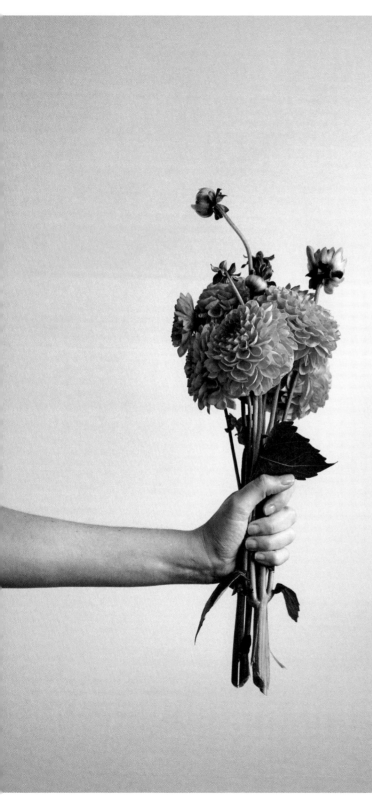

of the Inner Beauty ways I've been living into such celebrations, and I've found these extra touches of the sacred have been warmly received. Turning my make-up station into an Inner and Outer Beauty sanctuary, as well as layering in certain rituals and meditations, I found that I could add a sense of calm and connectedness into what could sometimes be anxious or busy preparations.

When some of my friends started to ask me to bring Inner Beauty rituals to their own celebrations, at first I felt a little hesitant. Leading a circle, as opposed to being one-on-one behind the scenes in my make-up work, was out of my normal comfort zone. But, dealing with a few nerves was totally worthwhile, as with each ritual we all felt our hearts embrace on a deeper level of celebration. So, here are some of my favourite rituals, which I've used in different moments of celebration.

'Many of the celebrations we know today traditionally have a deeper spiritual significance.'

Bride-to-be Ceremony

The idea of women gathering together before a wedding to celebrate the bride-to-be dates back at least to Ancient Greece. Women at this time had a specific ritual called a *Proaulia*, where the bride would spend her last days as a single woman with her mother, female relatives and friends. During these days, the bride would make sacred offerings to the gods and goddesses of love and the divine feminine, thanking them for protecting her childhood and marking her transition into adulthood. The offerings included old childhood toys, clothes and a lock of hair. These rituals would also strengthen adult bonds between the bride and the gods and goddesses who were needed to protect her in her transition to a new home and in creating a new family life.

The term 'hen party' actually originated in the 1800s as a term to describe gatherings of women for a cup of tea and a natter. But it wasn't until more recent times that the gathering of the hens became a key part of most wedding plans. For my own hen do, it was important for me to have a sacred dimension alongside all the usual fun and frolics. I invited one of my best friends to create a goddess ceremony. This was such a beautiful experience for me that I really wanted to share this gift with my other friends at their own hen dos. And so, I've found myself over the last few years holding the space for some really magical goddess ceremonies. These ceremonies are really a wonderful container in which we can celebrate the amazing qualities of the bride in a deeper way. I'm going to share a few ideas from these experiences with you now.

Preparation

If you are the person organizing the ceremony, you'll need to source a few things in advance. You need a bag of dried rose petals. You can either dry the petals yourself from your own rose plant, or you can buy them easily online. You'll also need some mini corked glass bottles/vials. One long necklace is required and you should ask each of the hens to bring a charm to thread onto that necklace during the ceremony (the charms can be anything that can be threaded on, from a stone or shell with a hole, or some pendant or charm you already had and wanted to gift). A beautiful centrepiece is essential, so bring a bowl, candles, crystals, photos of the couple, childhood photos of the bride-to-be, sacred sound

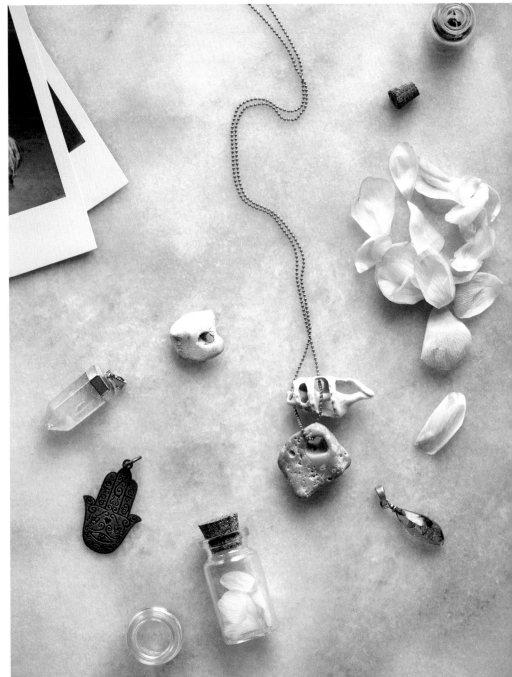

instruments (or even better if one of the hens plays a portable musical instrument, get her to bring this), and some incense and oils. Before the ceremony, give each of the hens a different Inner Beauty quality so they can write a short blessing for the bride which will be shared in circle (you can just email them beforehand so they have a little time to think). When you are ready to prepare the sacred space, fill the bowl with the rose petals and place it in the centre of the circle, arranging the other sacred objects around this bowl in a mindful and of course beautiful way.

Open the circle

Ideally, this ceremony is held on the morning of the hen do, so that everyone is relatively clear-headed before the corks are popped and the bubbles start flowing. As the person holding the ceremony, you will cleanse each hen as they enter into the circle, and give them one of the mini bottles. Once everyone is gathered and sat comfortably, it can be nice to ask people to close their eyes and guide them into a gentle meditation, taking a few deep breaths, connecting to their hearts and allowing some quiet space to mark the transition from hen chitter chatter to sacred time. (As the organizer, it's important you can drop into a place of peace and presence. It's OK to be a bit nervous, but taking a few quiet moments to connect and compose yourself before the ceremony begins can really help.) Using a sacred sound instrument can also help mark the transition from the excitable chitter chatter into this special ceremony. At this point, whilst people's eyes are still closed, you can ask the hens to hold their palms out. You will then walk around adding a couple of drops of your chosen oil blend into each outstretched palm. Then gently guide them to cup their hands over their noses, allowing the fragrant notes to connect them to a space of Inner Beauty.

Sharing blessings

At this point, the hens will take turns to share their Inner Beauty blessing for the bride, or bride and groom. Pass the necklace around, and as each hen speaks their blessing, they will thread the charm onto the necklace as a beautiful reminder of their words. To finish off this part of the ceremony, place the necklace around the neck of the bride-to-be. It is a love-filled coronation that is worthy of a goddess.

Rose petal reminders

To complete the ceremony, the bowl filled with rose petals is passed around, and each hen will take her mini bottle and fill this with the love-infused petals. This rose petal reminder is the perfect message-in-a-bottle to place in their sacred space or dressing table, reminding them of all the beautiful memories made that day.

♥ **Extra touch**

This ritual can also be translated into a birthday celebration ritual.

'I've found myself over the last few years holding the space for some really magical goddess ceremonies. These ceremonies are really a wonderful container in which we can celebrate the amazing qualities of the bride in a deeper way.'

Wedding Ritual

∞

For many women, a wedding day is the ultimate celebration, a culmination of years of dreaming about one day becoming a beautiful bride. To be honest, I never pictured myself having a big celebration in a big puffy, white dress, especially because the thought of being the centre of attention made me anxious. But, as the planning of my own wedding unfolded, I realized it's virtually impossible to do a Jewish wedding on a small scale, so I simply had to surrender. I was so glad I did, because it turned out to be the best day of my life.

One of my favourite parts was weaving Inner Beauty rituals throughout the day. A memory is now firmly etched into my heart of standing in ceremony with my husband in the middle of a circle of friends and family, feeling embraced by the love of everyone. We invited people at one stage in the ceremony to step forward and offer a blessing if they felt moved to. The spontaneity of this was really exciting, not having a clue what was coming, and we were awestruck when two of our beloved friends, Matt and Sally, stepped forward with their baby girl Phoebe in hand and broke into Carole King's 'You've got a friend'. Slowly but surely everyone started to join in and, by the end of the song, tears were running and hearts were broken wide open. The following are some extra sacred touches you might want to use or share with friends for a wedding-day celebration.

The night before

Excitement and nerves before The Big Day can make it hard to get enough beauty sleep. It can really help to create a sanctuary in the room where you're sleeping: a special bridal sacred space. In here, you can add another dimension of Inner Beauty to traditions such as the old British custom of having something old, something new, something borrowed, something blue. Something old signifies connection to the past, so this can, of course, be a special crystal (good love stones for weddings would be Rose Quartz, Rhodochrosite, Morganite and Apophyllite). Something new symbolizes optimism for the future, so why not treat yourself to a luxurious candle. Something borrowed relates to how happiness is shared with friends and family, so it might be a sacred object someone has lent you, a special piece of jewellery, a lucky charm. Something blue represents loyalty and purity, so a soft blue flower adds a really nice touch of beauty and calming energy to the bridal sacred space. Hydrangeas are a good choice: according to Doreen Virtue, as these flowers change colours from year to year, they offer symbolic support for a smooth transition.

Of course, the bride will have so much going on anyway that this can be a beautiful task to offer to one of the bridesmaids. It can be really relaxing as well to use some of the ideas from the earlier chapters on nurturing, bath-time and beauty sleep rituals. Cleansing takes on a particular importance the night before a wedding, as the bride wants to feel like she is entering into her wedding day free from any heavy energies of the past or with a little less of the nervous energy that has undoubtedly been building up. And the bedtime gratitude practice can be deepened on this special night by writing a letter to your future self a year from now. The first anniversary is paper, and so it's really nice to have a letter from yourself which has in it your dreams of where you'd like to see your relationship a year from now, where you see yourself living, what you see yourself doing, what advice you want to give to yourself, and simply sharing how you feel in this moment. The husband-to-be can do this too, so that you open them together on your anniversary.

The wedding morning

As a make-up artist, I've probably been at more wedding mornings than most, so I know what a whirlwind this time can be. If possible, it can really help to take even just a mindful minute to yourself. A really beautiful idea to help you stay connected to your calm centre when there are lots of people buzzing around is to add Inner Beauty tools to your dressing table: Rose Quartz and Blue Lace Agate crystals (both good for calming energy) and an oil-burner with some calming oils (neroli, pink lotus and rose mixed together work really well here).

At some recent weddings I've been involved in, I created a simple ritual, bringing a handful of Rose Quartz tumble stones to give to each of the bridesmaids and the mother of the bride, asking them to find a quiet, peaceful moment at some point during the morning when they could hold the stone and speak a blessing of love for the couple into it. The stones are then given back to the bride one-on-one, with each bridesmaid sharing her special blessing. The Maid of Honour is usually the best person to organize this small, simple ritual (don't forget to cleanse the stones before giving them to the bridesmaids). By the end of this process, the bride has all the love and support of her goddesses surrounding her on her dressing table. This collection of crystal blessings can be something the bride keeps on her dressing table beyond the wedding day too.

♥ Extra touches for your wedding ceremony

Through the Colourful Dot (my online Inner Beauty sanctuary), I've had the opportunity a few times in the last two years to provide crystal tumble stones for wedding rituals involving all of the guests. I get so excited when people ask me to do this. I just love to see more and more people wanting to sprinkle a little crystal magic throughout such a special day. One way people are using these tumble stones is really just an extension of the bridesmaid ritual above, where all guests are handed a tumble stone upon arriving at the ceremony. At one point, the celebrant asks everyone to take the crystal in hand, close their eyes, and put their highest wishes and blessings for the couple into the stone. Then somebody collects all the stones into a beautiful jar which will be not only a beautiful decoration to adorn the marital home, but also a powerful reminder and container of all the special wishes and intentions of their beloved friends and family.

Sunbeams

'A person who has good thoughts cannot ever be ugly. You can have a wonky nose and a crooked mouth and a double chin and stick-out teeth, but if you have good thoughts it will shine out of your face like sunbeams and you will always look lovely.'[10]

Roald Dahl, *The Twits*

10

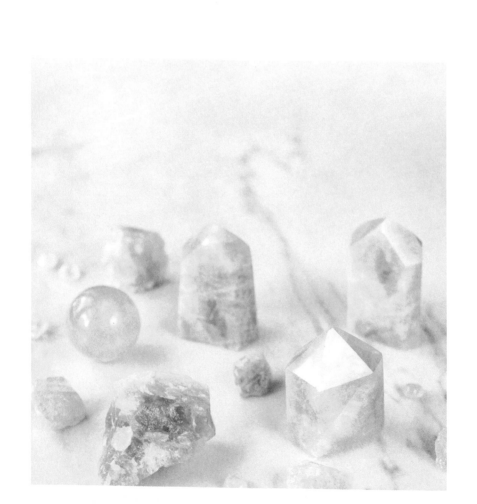

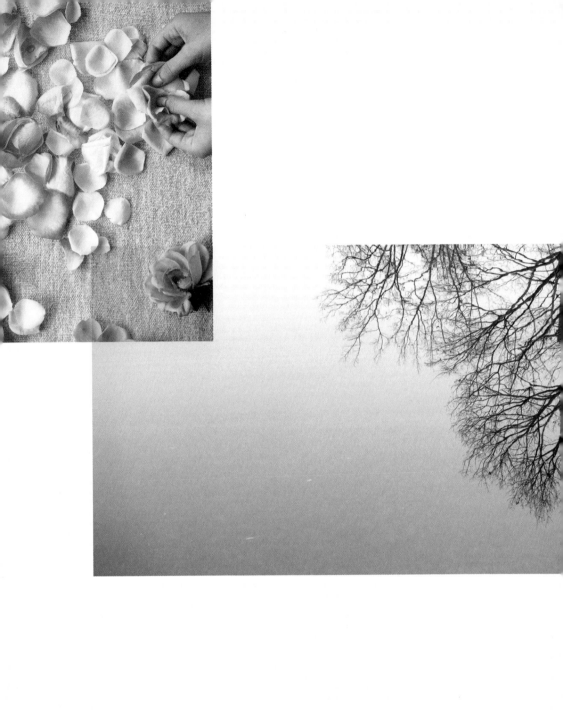

Thank you so much for taking the time to pick up this book. Whether you've read it from cover to cover, flicked through a couple of pages or even just enjoyed some of the images, I really hope that you've felt inspired to weave some Inner Beauty magic into your own daily life.

It's not easy to stay connected to our Inner Beauty. Having good thoughts singing out like sunbeams from our faces can feel impossible sometimes. We are human beings after all – the world affects us, leaves an imprint on our hearts. My hope is that this book will help us all to remember that there is a deeper beauty lying beneath the cracks; that only when we begin to acknowledge and embrace our imperfections can this beauty shine most brightly.

Special crystals are hidden deep in the earth. It takes time to find these crystals. Once one is found, time and energy is required to clean all the dirt away and polish the stone so that its natural beauty can radiate. In the same way, it takes time, energy and, above all, patience as we travel on this journey together, seeking to polish our hearts so that our true natural beauty can radiate out into the world. But in those moments when we do shine, when we really can feel that we are coming from a place of genuine love and we see the beautiful impact we can have on the world, in those moments we know that Inner Beauty is worth our efforts.

In rituals, we create a special moment where we give our Inner Beauty qualities the attention they need to grow. Without this special attention, they can remain hidden from view, just like the crystal hidden in the dirt.

We all desire deep down to see a world filled with more kindness. My hope for anyone reading this book – myself included – is that we can use the magic of Inner Beauty rituals to be just a little kinder to each other, and a little kinder to ourselves.

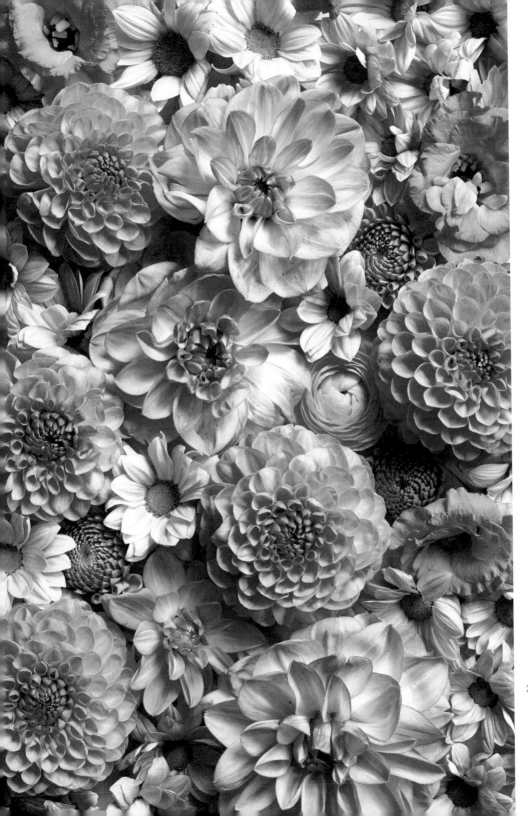

Index

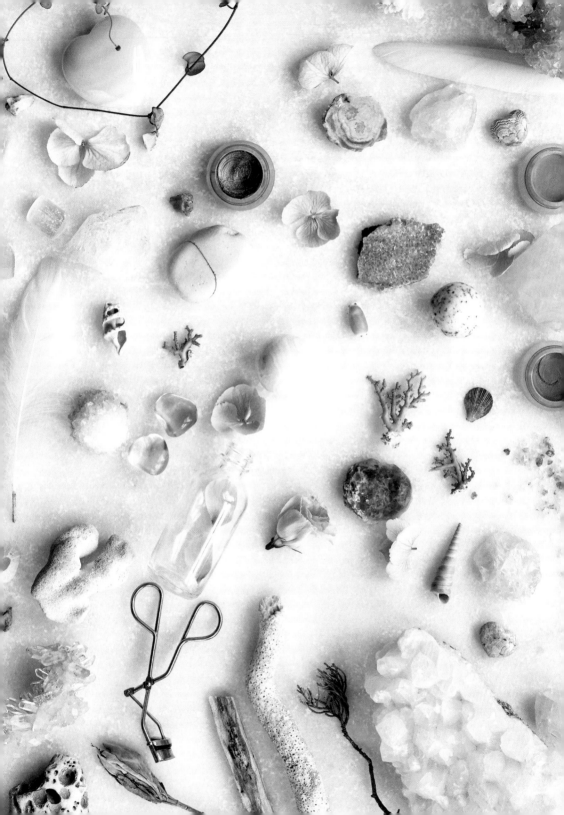

Endnotes

1. Ulrich, R. 'View through a window may influence recovery from surgery', *Science*, New Series, vol. 224, issue 4647 (April 27, 1984), pp. 420–1.

2. Weingarten, G. 'Pearls before breakfast: can one of the nation's great musicians cut through the fog of a D.C. rush hour?', *The Washington Post* (April 8, 2007).

3. Hongratanaworakit, T. 'Relaxing effect of rose oil on humans', *Natural Product Communications*, vol. 4, no. 2 (February 2009), pp. 291–6.

4. Mohagheghzadeh, A., Faridi, P., Shams-Ardakani, M., Ghasemi, Y. 'Medicinal smokes', *Journal of Ethnopharmacology*, vol. 108, issue 2 (24 November 2006), pp. 161–84.

5. Wolverton, B., Johnson, A., Bounds, K. 'Interior landscape plants for indoor air pollution abatement', *NASA* (September 15, 1989).

6. Dahl, Roald. *The Minpins*, published by Jonathan Cape Ltd and Penguin Books Ltd., 1991.

7. Bosch. 'House Moves and DIY projects' (22 June 2012).

8. *Nurses' Health Study* (1991).

9. Zheng, M., Fehr, R., Tai, K., Narayanan, J., Gelfand, M. 'The unburdening effects of forgiveness: effects on slant perception and jumping height', *Social Psychological and Personality Science*, vol. 6 (2015), pp. 431–8.

10. Dahl, Roald. *The Twits*, published by Jonathan Cape Ltd and Penguin Books Ltd., 1980.

—◇—

WITH
GRATITUDE TO
MOTHER EARTH
FOR HER
ABUNDANCE,
FOR HER
BEAUTY AND
FOR THE
WISDOM SHE
REVEALS.

—◇—

Acknowledgements

Wow, what a beautiful, emotional, challenging and inspiring journey it has been, writing this book. This creation could never have come into form without my lovely twin flame and hubby, Louis Weinstock, who helped me to write it, weaving his wisdom throughout this whole book. You have been my constant teacher – helping me to polish the mirror of my own heart and allowing my own inner beauty to shine, so I can be a more loving wife, daughter, sister, friend and hopefully mother one day soon.

Thank you to my family for always allowing me to express who I am.

Thank you to Rob and Sariet for showing me grace and strength in the face of adversity.

Thank you for all those who agreed to look at and critique parts of the book and for generally supporting us: Debbie Manning, Anne Weinstock, Rob Stewart, Kathleen Prior, Jo Bennett, Jenny Newmarch and Stephanie Sian Smith.

Thank you to my publisher, Carolyn Thorne, for giving me this precious opportunity, and to all the inspirational team at HarperCollins for adding your own special touches of beauty into this book: Melissa Okusanya, Lucy Sykes-Thompson and Isabel Hayman-Brown. Thank you also to Nassima Rothacker and Cynthia Blackett for the stunning images.

Thank you to our agent, Valeria Huerta, for supporting us along the way with determination and love.

Thank you to all those who shared their time and wisdom with me – with special mention to Suzanne Inayat-Khan, Nigel Hamilton, Roger Calverley, Carmen Sandoval, Maestra Martina Mamani, Elder Juan Gabriel Apaza Lonasco, Caroline Putnam and Sandra Pepper.

Thank you to all those teachers who have inspired me over the years, especially Mother Nature/Pachamama, who is my greatest teacher.

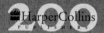

Thorsons
An imprint of HarperCollins*Publishers*
1 London Bridge Street
London SE1 9GF

www.harpercollins.co.uk

First published by Thorsons 2017

10 9 8 7 6 5 4 3 2

Text © Laurey Simmons 2016

Photography © Nassima Rothacker with the exception of the
    following: p38 (centre), p154 (middle), p155 (right), p199 (middle)
    © Laurey Simmons. p199 (centre) © Stephanie Sian Smith.
Prop stylist: Cynthia Blackett

A catalogue record of this book is available from
the British Library

ISBN 978-0-00-819674-5

Printed and bound in China

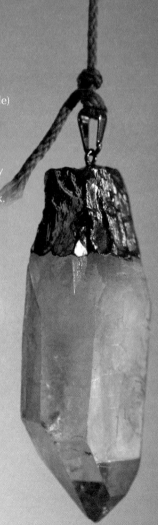